# The Post-Pregnancy
# Handbook

# THE
# POST-PREGNANCY
# HANDBOOK

The *Only* Book
That Tells What the
First Year After Childbirth
Is *Really* All About—
Physically, Emotionally,
Sexually

❖ ❖ ❖

## SYLVIA BROWN

*with Mary Dowd Struck, R.N., M.S., C.N.M.*

ILLUSTRATIONS BY
CHRISTIANE SCHAEFFER

St. Martin's Griffin 🐾 New York 🅼

ILLUSTRATIONS BY CHRISTIANE SCHAEFFER

Library of Congress Cataloging-in-Publication Data

Brown, Sylvia.
 The post-pregnancy handbook : The only book that tells what the first year
after childbirth is really all about—physically, emotionally, sexually /
Sylvia Brown with Mary Dowd Struck.
  p. cm.
 ISBN 0-312-30064-6 (hc)
 ISBN 0-312-31626-7 (pbk)
 1. Postnatal care—Handbooks, manuals, etc. 2. Motherhood—
Handbooks, manuals, etc. 3. Childbirth—Handbooks, manuals, etc.
4. Infants—Care—Handbooks, manuals, etc. I. Struck, Mary Dowd. II. Title.

RG801 .B76 2002
618.6—dc21                                                      2001057897

First published under the title *Le guide de l'après-accouchement* in France
by Bibliothèque de la famille, Éditions Albin Michel, 2000.

10  9  8  7  6  5  4  3  2

*For Adrian and Laure,*
*who have made it all worthwhile*

# Contents

**Introduction**                                           xiii

**Classical Medications and Alternative Remedies**           1
Classical Medications                                        1
Alternative Remedies                                         2
*Homeopathy*                                                 4
*Herbal Remedies*                                            6
*Acupuncture and Chinese Medicine*                           8
*Manual Therapies*                                          10

## I ✦ THE FIRST FEW DAYS

1.  **A Great Physical Upheaval**                           19
    The Hormonal Revolution                                 20
    The Reproductive System                                 22
    The Recovery Process                                    23

2.  **Caring for the Genital Organs**                        28
    The Uterus                                               28
    The Birth Canal                                          31
    After an Episiotomy                                      33

3.  **Your Bodily Functions After Childbirth**               42
    Urination                                                42
    Fluid Retention                                          44
    The Digestive Tract                                      45
    Your First Exercises After Childbirth                    49

4.  **Coping with the Side Effects of Childbirth**           52
    The Common Side Effects of Childbirth                    52
    Circulatory Problems                                     57
    Hemorrhoids                                              58
    After an Epidural                                        62

5.  **After a Cesarean Section**                             67
    The Operation                                            67
    Discomfort After a Cesarean                              70
    The Baby Born by Cesarean                                76

6.  **Reclaiming Your Body**                                 78
    Rehabilitating the Pelvic Floor Muscles                  79
    Recovering Pelvic Balance                                80

7.  **Possible Postpartum Complications**                    84
    Infections                                               84
    Hemorrhages                                              88
    Serious Circulatory Problems                             90

## II ✦ YOUR FIRST FEW WEEKS

8.  **A Changed Lifestyle**                                  95
    Your Fragile Body                                        95
    Getting Your Routine Under Control                       97

Organizing Your Return Home                                 100
Relationships Change                                              104
Surviving Fatigue                                                   110

9.  Looking After Your Body                                     114
    Your Posture                                                      114
    Exercises for the First Six Weeks After Childbirth     119
    Hygiene                                                             121
    Bleeding                                                           121
    Healing Your Scars                                              123
    Infections                                                          124
    Your Appearance                                                126

10. Diet After Childbirth                                           134
    The Impact of Childbirth                                        134
    How to Get What You Need                                    135
    Your Dietary Habits                                              139
    A Word About Dieting                                            140

11. Resuming Your Menstrual Cycle                             142
    Your First Period After Childbirth                             142
    Your Fertility                                                       142
    The Postnatal Visit                                                145

12. Returning to Work                                               147
    Breast-feeding for the Working Mother                      149

III ✦ BREAST-FEEDING

13. Common Myths About Breast-feeding                      153
    The Importance of a Good Start                               154
    The Truth Behind the Myths                                    155

14. Breast-feeding: Getting Off to a Good Start            159
    How the Breasts Produce Milk                                 159
    The Golden Rules                                                  161

The Feed   165

Breast-feeding Problems   172

Mother's Milk for Premature or Sick Babies   183

15. **An Established Routine**   185

Integrating Breast-feeding into Your Routine   186

Weaning   188

16. **The Nursing Mother's Diet**   190

The Basics   191

## IV ✦ EMOTIONAL REACTIONS TO CHILDBIRTH

17. **The First Days**   197

A Time of Change   197

Your First Encounter with the Baby   199

Communicating with the Newborn   202

Caring for the Baby   205

The Never-ending Story of Childbirth   206

Special Cases   207

"Baby Blues"   210

18. **Emotional Reactions of the First Few Months**   216

Overcoming Mild Depression   217

Managing Stress   226

19. **Postnatal Depression**   233

Symptoms of Postnatal Depression   234

The Causes of Postnatal Depression   235

Healing the Mind   238

Puerperal Psychosis   242

20. **The Mother in You**   243

Maternal Instinct: Is It in All of Us?   243

The "Perfect Mother"   244

The Impact of Our Families   248

Raising a Child                                                          251
Lack of Recognition                                                     255
Expectations Management                                                 257

## V ✦ THE COUPLE

21. **The Couple Changes**                                              261
    When a Woman Becomes a Mother                                       262
    When a Man Becomes a Father                                         265
    Father and Child                                                    268
    Common Stumbling Blocks                                             271

22. **A Little Patience: Sex After Childbirth**                         274
    Physical Impediments to Sexual Desire                               274
    Psychological Obstacles to Sexual Desire                            275
    Reclaiming Your Intimacy                                            277

## VI ✦ A FULL RECOVERY

23. **First Things First: The Pelvic Floor**                            283
    The Importance of the Pelvic Floor                                  283
    Lift and Squeeze: A Brief Review of Pelvic Floor Anatomy            285
    What Affects the Pelvic Floor Muscles?                              287
    Urogenital Problems                                                 290
    Urinary Incontinence                                                291
    Anal Leakage                                                        293
    Organ Prolapse                                                      293
    Toning and Strengthening the Pelvic Floor                           296

24. **A New Body Image**                                                300
    Your Weight                                                         300
    Exercise                                                            304
    Posture and Your Back                                               309

**Acknowledgments**                                                     317
**Index**                                                               319

# Introduction

By my fourteenth shower of the day, I became truly angry: Why was I so sore? No one had warned me that the days following childbirth could be so painful. I had attended prenatal classes, endlessly discussed the topic with my girlfriends, read a good dozen books on pregnancy and childcare. Not one had hinted that my insides might feel like they had been scraped with a cheese grater, nor that hemorrhoids could hurt so much, nor that it would be impossible to find a comfortable position, even lying down. I was in a prestigious maternity hospital but no one offered me the slightest tip or nonmedical remedy to alleviate all these aches and pains (I discovered the wonderfully soothing effect of running water all on my own—which explains my seventeen showers on the second day). To make matters worse, the midwife for whom I most cared was on a training course, and my doctor had left town immediately after my delivery to attend a family wedding. So there was not much sympathy coming from these quarters.

Once home, I found myself alone (my husband, a United Nations official, was posted at the time in the Balkans during the Yugoslav war and returned to work the day after our son was born), without a mother or mother-in-law, in an unfamiliar city (I had decided to have the baby in Paris, which was closer than the U.S. to our posting). As a result, I did not have the all-important "support network" which I discuss at length later in this book. Just like many other new mothers, I did not think that my discomfort warranted disturbing my obstetrician. The few pages on the postnatal period contained in various pregnancy handbooks seemed to gloss over these issues with a sweeping ". . . everything will be fine within a few days." This is when I decided to write my own guide to the days and weeks following childbirth, a book for mothers by a mother, filled with practical advice and realistic solutions.

I began by mentioning the idea to my doctor: "You're a wonderful obstetrician, but your postnatal care leaves something to be desired . . . I therefore need your assistance in undertaking a project whose aim is to help women better understand their body, know when to seek medical advice, and thus take control of their health." He responded enthusiastically and gave me bountifully of a doctor's most precious asset: his time.

Having spent ten years working in financial marketing, my second task was to take a survey of my future readers by distributing an anonymous questionnaire to 300 new mothers. Their answers confirmed the statistics I had seen in medical journals: 64 percent of women have bad memories of their postnatal experience. Furthermore, 47 percent of new mothers have at least one health concern in the six weeks after childbirth (back pain, migraines, and urinary incontinence, to mention but a few). In two-thirds of these cases, the problem persists well past the traditional postpartum phase. Indeed, pregnancy and childbirth have the unfortunate effect of revealing certain dormant health problems, or of exacerbating existing conditions.

Thanks to my dual Franco-American nationality, I was able to conduct research on both sides of the Atlantic. Over the course of three years, fifty-five specialists shared their knowledge and experience with me. The *Post-Pregnancy Handbook* was originally published in 2000 in France, where I had myself given birth to my two children. It has now been completely rewritten to meet American medical standards and has been adapted for the U.S. market. Before undertaking this rather awesome editing job, I was extremely fortunate to meet Mary Dowd Struck, head nurse at the Women and Infants Hospital in Providence, Rhode

Island, which is not only one of America's top maternity hospitals but also at the forefront of innovation in obstetric practice.

In almost all non-Western cultures, the postnatal period is viewed as a time of healing, rest, and recuperation accompanied by specific rituals and traditions. Regardless of the actual effectiveness of these customs, they have the merit of making the new mother feel cherished and cared for at a time of great physical and emotional vulnerability. Such a sense of support will almost inevitably accelerate the recovery process. Most of these rituals also underscore the fact that recovering from childbirth takes time—forty days of complete rest in an almost exclusively female environment is common to many cultures. Our great-grandmothers and, for some, grandmothers, stayed in bed for twenty-one days. In 1970, the normal hospital stay in the United States was four days. By 1990, it was down to twenty-four hours. Since the passage of the Family and Medical Leave Act, it is now forty-eight hours for a normal delivery, and ninety-six hours after a cesarean section. But the length of hospital stay is only half the issue: the real problem in Western societies today is the lack of help and support for the new mother when she returns home. We so often hear that pregnancy and childbirth are not an illness that we no longer recognize the enormous physical and mental effort required to bring a child into the world.

At the beginning of the twentieth century, a woman had a 10 percent chance of dying each time she gave birth. Childbirth was the second most common cause of death after tuberculosis. Today, we take it for granted that we will leave the maternity hospital completely unscathed. Prenatal diagnostic tools, IVF, and epidural anesthesia all give us a completely different perception of childbirth than our predecessors had. We now have the luxury to experience childbirth as an enriching event and to focus above all on the welfare of the baby. As a result, we have tended to forget to take care of ourselves.

Since our expectations are now much higher than those of preceding generations were, we also run a greater risk of experiencing frustration and deception. We think that we can integrate a baby into a professional life that has been highly structured for many years. We expect our partners instantly to become perfect fathers and we begin immediately judging them on their ability to change a diaper or give a bath. Most of all, we refuse to accept that the postnatal period is a state of transition at all levels. The arrival of a child will change our lives forever, and adjusting to this reality takes time.

Far too many women have bad memories of their "tenth month." What a pity! There seems to exist a kind of secrecy around the subject, as if no one dared admit that this transitional phase could be difficult. And yet medical advances in the post-pregnancy phase are impressive. A well-informed woman who understands what is happening to her body has every reason to live through a positive experience.

Most women feel highly motivated to take better care of themselves through their pregnancy. They generally actively seek information and undergo regular medical supervision. But if they really stop to think about their changes in lifestyle, most future mothers will admit that they are concerned primarily with the health of their baby. . . . Recovering from childbirth is a unique opportunity for women to think about themselves and permanently adopt healthy habits in their nonpregnant state as well. This means understanding your body, knowing how to identify its alarm bells, eating a healthy diet, exercising appropriately, and watching your posture.

We all have been exposed to images of the "joys of motherhood" to such an extent that new mothers fear to discuss their problems and simply "grin and bear it." Yet, there are so many remedies and solutions available. How can you alleviate discomfort? What precautionary measures should you take? How can you understand what you are feeling? How do you know if medical assistance is required? Throughout this book, we will give you advice and tips on how to live through a better post-pregnancy experience. We will point out serious problems that require immediate medical attention. And, in addition to classical medical remedies, we will suggest treatments from a range of alternative practices such as homeopathy, aromatherapy, plant therapy, Chinese medicine, and manual therapies.

In order to be genuinely loving and committed to our children, we must experience our own sense of well-being and satisfaction. Taking time to care for ourselves physically and emotionally is the greatest contribution we can make to our families.

# The Post-Pregnancy Handbook

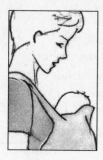

# Classical Medications and Alternative Remedies

## Classical Medications

During your hospital stay and while recuperating at home, you may be prescribed various types of classical medications. These generally fall into the following categories: anti-inflammatories, analgesics, antibiotics, and uterotonics.

Anti-inflammatory drugs such as ibuprofen (Advil, Motrin, Excedrin IB, etc.) or acetaminophen (Tylenol) are used to reduce swelling and discomfort. NSAIDs, as they are called, should be taken with a full glass of water or milk with meals to reduce gastric irritation, a possible side effect of these drugs.

Narcotic analgesics are used to treat moderate to severe pain. Women use them most often after a cesarean birth. Percocet or Tylenol with codeine are the most frequently prescribed.

Antibiotics are used to treat infections. The most common sites for infections after childbirth are the urinary tract and the uterus, as will be described on pages 84 to 87.

Uterotonics are a class of drugs that cause the uterus to contract. The most common are oxytocin (Pitocin, the same drug used to induce labor), and methergine. They are prescribed if the uterus is not contracting well after delivery or if the woman is bleeding heavily.

Stool softeners or laxatives, particularly Colace and mineral oil, are used to prevent or treat constipation. You should ask your nurse for a stool softener if you have an uncomfortable episiotomy or are taking narcotic analgesics that could cause constipation.

There are many other drugs used to treat specific problems that occur as a result of pregnancy or delivery. Whenever your doctor prescribes a medication, please be sure to ask him/her the purpose of the drug and its common side effects.

## Alternative Remedies

Recent studies in both the Unites States and Great Britain show an explosion of interest in alternative remedies (also known as complementary medicine). As consumers increasingly demand to be more actively involved in medical decisions, alternative therapies give patients the opportunity to act in partnership with their health care professionals. Alternative remedies are based on a holistic view of health care where body, mind, and spirit all have equal importance. Ill health is a due to a disharmony within the whole person and is shown by the symptoms expressed. Each person is viewed as an individual in the wider context of his or her environment. While conventional medicine is aimed at reacting to and suppressing symptoms as they arise, alternative remedies seek to promote prevention and to assist the body's own defense mechanism. Indeed, the body's innate ability to heal itself forms the starting point for all the major alternative approaches to medicine.

A number of alternative therapies are particularly appropriate during pregnancy and the postnatal period when many health problems result from adjustment difficulties. It is therefore important to stimulate the body toward a new equilibrium by working with its natural processes in a gentle and harmonious manner.

In the months surrounding childbirth when most drugs and conventional medications are proscribed, remedies such as homeopathy and herbs are for the most part harmless and nontoxic. Their use promotes a "self-help" attitude which puts a woman at the center of her own experience and permits her to take back control of her body at a time when she may feel particularly vulnerable. Since the patient is as much responsible for involvement in the treatment as the therapist, a fair measure of self-awareness is required to use alternative remedies, and thus they provide an excellent way for a mother to remain "in touch" with her body after pregnancy and childbirth.

Alternative therapies can claim success in treating a wide range of conditions, particularly chronic complaints. They also work extremely well when used in conjunction with conventional medications. But they should never be used at the expense of normal midwifery or obstetric practice. Always remember that where a remedy has the power to do good, it also has the potential to do harm if used inappropriately or inaccurately. Practitioners must be adequately and appropriately trained (it is preferable that they have a strong background in conventional medicine). As with all medication, some women may react differently to specific cures.

Alternative remedies work just as rapidly as classical medications. They may even help the body fight viruses by reinforcing its natural defenses.

Until recently, research on alternative therapies was either not published or improperly written up. It is now appearing in mainstream medical journals—with the caveat, however, that double-blind, randomized clinical trials are not always appropriate methodology for complementary medical research.

More than 140 different alternative therapies have been catalogued. Five, however, are nationally regulated in many western countries, with codes of conduct and defined criteria for education and training. These are: homeopathy, osteopathy, chiropracy, acupuncture, and medical herbalism. Another five therapies can act in a supportive role when used alongside conventional or other complementary treatments. These are: aromatherapy, massage, reflexology, shiatsu/acupressure, and hypnotherapy.

In her book *Alternative Therapies for Pregnancy and Birth*, Patricia Thomas reminds us of the following guidelines when using alternative remedies:

◆ Alternative remedies are not magic or talismans. Their ingredients are not trade secrets. You should be able to understand how each works and what it is supposed to do.

◆ Treatments should not hurt. You should not go through a prolonged "healing crisis" (aggravated symptoms or unpleasant
  side effects).

◆ It may take longer to address a cause than simply to suppress
  a symptom. Don't bounce from one remedy to another simply
  because things are not moving fast enough.

◆ Less is more—you need only take a remedy until you feel better since the treatment supports the body's ability to heal and
  change, not to undermine or replace.

◆ Work with your body; "tune in." Observe appropriate lifestyle
  and dietary habits to support your treatment.

## Homeopathy

The word *homeopathy* comes from the Greek *homois*, meaning "similar,"
and *pathos*, meaning "suffering." Homeopathic remedies are infinitesimal
doses of medicine derived from a variety of plant, mineral, chemical, and
animal sources which are ingested (generally as small white pills) to
enhance the body's own capacity for both physical and emotional healing. This approach is based on the idea that "like cures like." While
orthodox medicine uses opposites—for example, in the case of constipation, a medicine will be given which produces diarrhea—homeopathy
uses similars—for example, a remedy known to produce constipation in
crude form would cure the constipation if given in a small dose.

The Law of Similars was well known to the ancient Greeks. In 1790,
it was resurrected by a German physician, Samuel Hahnemann, in reaction to the barbaric medical practices of his time. He spent his life
developing and cataloguing over two thousand relationships between
diseases and their symptoms, as well as the toxic effects of natural
medically active substances.

Homeopathic remedies are so diluted that no molecules of the original substance remain. Most commonly used is the centennial scale
where one part of the remedy is diluted with 99 parts of water or alcohol, then shaken. The number following the names of the homeopathic
remedy indicates how many times this process has occurred. For example, Arnica 6C means that the medicine was diluted, shaken, then
diluted again six times. Incredibly, the more times the dilution process
occurs, the more potent the medicine! The apparent explanation for
this phenomenon is that the process of dilution and shaking imprints

the characteristic energy pattern or blueprint of the original substance onto the water in which it is diluted.

Homeopathy has received considerable medical scrutiny in recent years. A 1997 article in the highly respected British medical journal *The Lancet* reviewed all properly conducted clinical trials between 1943 and 1995, finding that 77 percent of studies demonstrated that homeopathy yielded positive results and that homeopathy was ten times more effective than a placebo. It is nevertheless difficult to use classical scientific tests on homeopathy, as these require assembling a group of homogeneous persons with the same named disease. Since homeopathy does not recognize diseases but only diseased individuals, each person will be different and it will be impossible to create a homogeneous group.

Homeopathy is particularly well suited to pregnancy, childbirth, and the postpartum period as it produces no side effects and is nonaddictive. If the remedy is wrong, it simply will not work. Often, only a single dose is required. And when the desired change has occurred, no further medication is required.

One great advantage of homeopathy is that many basic remedies can be bought over-the-counter and be self-administered. They are indicated throughout this book. Simply remember the following guidelines:

- ✦ Do not touch the pills. Count them out into the bottle top and tip the contents into your mouth, letting the pills melt under your tongue.
- ✦ Avoid food for twenty minutes before or after taking a homeopathic remedy.
- ✦ Avoid mint, eucalyptus, camphor, cigarettes, and caffeine when undergoing a homeopathic treatment.

Any persistent or serious condition which does not improve within a week requires the advice of a homeopathic practitioner, preferably one who fully trained in classical medicine before further specializing in homeopathy. The practitioner will ask for a full medical history and study patterns of symptoms. Some may look for a single remedy to treat you constitutionally, while others will address symptom patterns with a combination of remedies.

While it is important to remember that homeopathy cannot repair irreversible damage and is no substitute for emergency surgery, it is particularly helpful in curing the following typical postnatal problems:

- ✦ *After pains*: Homeopathic remedies generally work within twenty-four hours to alleviate painful uterine contractions after childbirth (see pages 28–31). As opposed to many classical medications given in maternity hospitals, they do not contraindicate breast-feeding.
- ✦ *Episiotomies*: Homeopathic remedies have been shown to promote better healing. Pain generally disappears within three days.
- ✦ *Cesarean sections*: Using homeopathic remedies after a C-section helps the digestive system to recover much faster than with classical medication (normal passage of gas within twenty-four hours instead of two or three days; normal defecation within two days instead of four). Homeopathy can also help women who react badly to anesthesia and morphine.
- ✦ *Baby blues*: Homeopathic remedies work faster than classical medication to alleviate mild depressive symptoms (generally twenty-four hours instead of two days).

## Herbal Remedies

Plantlife has long been considered necessary to support human life. Herbal medicine was central to many ancient cultures and today many familiar medicines have been copied from natural blueprints: aspirin from white willow bark, morphine and codeine from opium poppies, quinine from the cinchona bark, antiulcer drugs from licorice.

There are two ways to approach herbal remedies: either to use the whole plant or to isolate only the active constituents in a plant. The followers of the first approach claim, to use the words of Denise Tiran and Sue Mack in *Complementary Therapies for Pregnancy and Childbirth*, "that the medicinal property ascribed to a particular herb is not that of a single active constituent but rather an orchestra of ingredients working synergistically and thereby reinforcing the overall positive effect of the herb." They also claim that the remedy will be better tolerated. Those who prefer distilling only the active ingredient in a plant point to the fact that extra cellulose and nonactive parts will make the remedy less potent and less well absorbed.

Herbal remedies can be taken internally or applied externally as ointments, creams, and essential oils. As they are very powerful, they should be used with the same caution and respect as any medication.

+ Internally, they can be ingested as infusions (fresh or dried leaves, flowers or stems steeped in boiling water); tinctures (concentrated drops derived from steeping raw herbs in water, vinegar, or alcohol); or capsules (modern extraction methods give us remedies thirty times more potent than old-fashioned dried plants).
+ Externally, plant extracts can be added to ointments and creams for topical application.

## Aromatherapy

Essential oils (which contain no oily substances!) are distilled and extracted from plants, flowers, trees, barks, grasses, and seeds. Each has a distinct chemical makeup and unique therapeutic, psychological, and physiological effect. The French chemist Rene Maurice Gattefosse pioneered their modern use in the 1930s and coined the term *aromatherapy*. Later, an Austrian biochemist, Marguerite Maury, began prescribing essential oils as remedies to her patients and was the first to use essential oils in massage. Studies have shown that inhaling fragrances can cause changes in both the circulation and electrical activity of the brain. Smell has the most direct connection to the mind and emotions since the nose has direct access to the limbic system (emotional switchboard of the brain). Fragrances may also be absorbed through the skin. The way an oil is used will enhance its effect on the body; with a massage, in a bath, by steam inhalation, in an oil burner, diffuser or vaporizer, or sprinkled on a pillow.

Since essential oils are so concentrated, very few are safe to use neat on skin and require dilution in a base or carrier oil, such as sweet almond oil, apricot kernel oil, grapeseed oil, safflower oil, or hazelnut oil. Beware of cheap or synthetic base oils that may inactivate the healing properties of the essential oils. These base oils can also be enriched by adding 10 percent of carrot, borrage seed, avocado, evening primrose, jojoba, wheat germ or sesame oil. A certain number of drops of essential oil are then added to a specific quantity of base. No more than five different essential oils should be mixed at one time.

In the postnatal period, aromatherapy is particularly useful for healing wounds (certain essential oils are excellent antiseptics, reduce swelling, and promote healthy scar tissue) and for alleviating emotional and hormonal problems.

Just as with homeopathy, many herbal remedies can be purchased in health food stores (supermarket herbal teas have almost no therapeutic value) and then self-administered. However, health practitioners with further training in medicinal herbs may provide valuable advice in case of persistent problems. Be sure to check a therapist's credentials to ensure that his or her training is not just in aromatherapy as a beauty treatment.

### Bach Flower Remedies

Bach Flower Remedies belong to a group of alternative remedies known as vibrational medicine. These are tinctures and essences that are charged with a particular frequency of subtle healing energy, particularly for emotional problems.

At the end of the nineteenth century, a British bacteriologist, Dr. Edward Bach, studied the healing properties of plant essences and identified thirty-eight healing remedies corresponding to thirty-eight negative states which influence the course of illness and well-being. These are commonly divided into two groups: "type remedies," referring to personality types, and "mood remedies," which refer to a person's present emotional state. A prescription of Bach Flower Remedies will be tailored to suit the patient's changing situation and their reaction at a particular point in time. The tinctures come in small bottles and are ingested either by placing the prescribed number of drops under the tongue or by pouring the drops in a small glass of water. These remedies are very gentle and present no known side effects. Bach Flower Remedies are found in many health food stores. More and more, naturalists and herbal medicine practitioners are trained in their prescription.

## Acupuncture and Chinese Medicine

In Chinese, the life energy that surrounds us and flows through us is called *Qi* or *Chi*. When this life force is disturbed either because it is blocked or because it is moving too slowly or too fast, imbalance and eventually illness will result. Acupuncture is a system of healing which aims to restore health by bringing life energy into balance.

Acupuncture is one of the principal healing methods of Chinese medicine. This three thousand-year-old science divides the universe into two systems of reference: the *Yin* principle, which corresponds to coldness, darkness, the interior, passiveness, and the negative, and the *Yang* principle, which implies warmth, light, activity, expressiveness, and the positive. In the body, Yin represents the architecture: bones, muscles, the circulatory system. Yang is the unconscious, the intellectual, and everything that moves inside the body's architecture. If either Yin or Yang becomes unbalanced, then health disorders will result.

Energy flows throughout our body along a system of channels known as meridians, which lie in the connective tissues that sheath the circulatory, nervous, muscular, skeletal, digestive and other major body systems. Every movement of the body creates bioelectric signals (energy) which run along the meridians, through the connective tissues, eventually ending up at the skin. Thus it is possible to touch a specific point on the skin and "send a message" to all the internal organs and tissues that are along the meridian. This explains why a weak liver can show up as leg cramps, a rash on the inner thighs, or a runny nose, as all these points are on the liver meridian. This is the underlying principle of acupuncture and shiatsu/acupressure.

Birth represents a brutal disruption in the body's natural equilibrium. During nine months, the baby and the amniotic fluid—both Yin elements—increased progressively. Suddenly, all this Yin energy disappears, causing blockages in the circulatory system, which result in many of the typical disorders of the postpartum period. The excess Yang energy disturbs the body on the emotional level, leading to depression. Chinese medicine can be used to restore the proper Yin/Yang equilibrium in the following ways:

+ Through diet, by eating primarily Yin foods such as proteins and warm drinks, and by minimizing Yang foods such as raw vegetables and milk products.
+ By breathing very deeply to massage the liver, the organ most affected by the hormonal changes and slower circulation of the postpartum.
+ By keeping the area around the kidneys as warm as possible (warm showers, a heating pad). In many Asian cultures, new mothers lie on special beds under which hot coals are placed at the level of the kidneys.

✦ By stimulating the meridians that will conduct Yin energy to the organs that most need it.

Acupuncture uses needles like small antennas to conduct energy from one of two thousand points on the body's surface to the organs and tissues inside. The needles are tiny and only penetrate the superficial layers of the skin. Sometimes, the therapist will increase the stimulation by also using finger pressure, massage, electricity, or heat in the form of a small cigar-shaped bundle of herbs know as moxa which is lit and held a short distance from the skin. This technique will boost the immune system, activate energy, treat disease, promote the body's natural healing powers, and alleviate fatigue. It is safe, effective, and gently nudges the body back into harmony.

Of all the alternative medical practices, acupuncture is the best researched and documented. The World Health Organization now states that there is sufficient medical evidence to support the effectiveness of acupuncture and for it to be considered an important part of primary health care. For example, a 1994 German study found that acupuncture was at least as effective as iron supplements in raising blood hemoglobin (iron levels).

In choosing a therapist, be sure to check the credentials of your practitioner, who should have three to five years training in acupuncture as well as a strong background in classical medicine. At the first appointment, you will be asked detailed questions on your lifestyle, diet, work, medical history, and emotional state. The therapist will examine your pulse and tongue, two important diagnostic tools in Chinese medicine. A maximum of five to eight needles should be used for the treatment—fifteen to twenty are far too many. And strict hygiene rules must be observed: disposable needles, clean hands, etc.

## Manual Therapies

Osteopathy and chiropractic science emerged in the West about one hundred years ago. Shiatsu comes to us from Japan and is derived from an ancient form of massage. All seek to permit an unhindered flow of energy through the body.

The spine is the bearer of the mother and her child. Some of the most profound changes experienced during pregnancy take place along the spine. Increased weight leads to greater curvatures, resulting in pain in the lower back, buttocks, and down the legs. The pelvis becomes unstable as the hormones of pregnancy soften its bones and ligaments in order to make them more flexible to allow the baby's passage. Labor itself is a tremendous strain on the hip joints and lumbar spine, especially if the mother gives birth in the lithotomy position (on her back with her feet in stirrups). Then, in the postnatal period, the new mother is subject to more bending and lifting than before, to the fatigue of altered sleep patterns, and often sits in a bad position while breast-feeding. Little wonder that more than 50 percent of pregnant and post-pregnant women experience back pain.

Since the spine is connected via multiple pathways to all the organs of the body, these disturbances may result in problems in other parts of the body. Not surprisingly, it has been found that treating back pain can cure other common problems of pregnancy.

## Osteopathy

Developed by an American engineer, Dr. Andrew Taylor Still, in the late 1800s, osteopathy is based on the principle that the body is a self-regulating, self-healing organism whose structure is directly related to its function. The aim of osteopathy (OMT—osteopathic manipulative therapy) is to preserve the balance between the muscles, joints, ligaments, and nerves so that the body can function effectively.

William Garner Sutherland refined Still's ideas and proved that the body is in a constant, dynamic state of motion. He also noted that our tissues and organs and bones have a unique pulse that expands and contracts in a harmonious rhythmic impulse. The musculoskeletal system influences the body through the nervous system; therefore, its function depends on the unhindered flow of nerve impulses (transporting essential cell substances and electricity), blood, and lymphatic fluids.

Osteopathic philosophy maintains that the structure and functions of the body are inseparable. Since problems in one organ affect other organ systems, manipulation has a distinct effect beyond the muscular-skeletal system.

During pregnancy, osteopathy can help with aches and pains, particularly back problems due to changes in posture as the body accommodates the increasing size and weight of the uterus. Many expectant mothers also have found osteopathy useful in reducing nausea, heartburn, breathing difficulties, and circulatory problems (especially varicose veins and hemorrhoids).

After childbirth, osteopathy is highly recommended to restore the body's alignment following the inevitable trauma of delivery. If the mother's coccyx (tailbone) has been displaced (as is the case in one in ten vaginal deliveries), an osteopath is urgently needed to alleviate the resulting back pain. Realigning the pelvis also is the necessary first step to curing postnatal urinary incontinence. Most important, restoring the balance of the body's various systems is essential to recovering energy after childbirth.

One specialized area of osteopathy, known as craniosacral osteopathy, attempts to regulate the flow of the cerebrospinal fluid that runs from the base of our skull to the tip of our spine. By gently manipulating areas of the upper neck and skull, the therapist can feel this pulse. As it is extremely precise and gentle, this form of osteopathy is particularly suitable for small babies who have been traumatized during a difficult delivery.

Osteopaths today are often also trained in soft tissue manipulation to help improve the flow of vital energy in the body. The technique is used to resolve digestive, low-energy, circulatory, and other organ problems.

Osteopathy is now well respected in many countries. In Great Britain, it is the only alternative therapy accorded the status of a statutorily self-regulated profession. In the 1960s, the American College of Osteopathy joined the medical establishment. A D.O. (doctor of osteopathy) is the equivalent of a M.D. (medical doctor).

As of April 2001, osteopathy was accepted by the Federation of State Medical Boards of the United States as being a complete and equal school of medicine to allopathy (conventional medicine). There are currently ninety colleges of osteopathic medicine in the U.S. and about 48,500 D.O.s, representing one in twenty physicians in the U.S. Unlike their counterparts in other countries, American D.O.s are licensed to render complete patient care including prescribing regulated pharmaceuticals and performing surgery.

Osteopathy differs from classical physiotherapy, which focuses mainly on the area causing the symptom and not on the body as a whole. However, many physiotherapists have chosen to further their studies by following a five-year course in osteopathy or chiropractic science.

## Chiropractic Science

Just as with osteopathy, chiropractic science is a manual therapy based on the concept that the body has an inherent ability to heal itself. "Chiropractic" comes from the Greek word *chiropraktikos*, meaning "effective treatment by hand." Like osteopaths, chiropractors use the relationship between the nervous system and the mechanical framework of the body to restore harmony and thus good health. Chiropractic science is, however, more concerned with the relative *position* of the joints (especially the spinal joints) rather than their relative mobility. Therefore the therapist often uses X ray to diagnose a problem and focuses primarily on the spine to evaluate structure and function. The chiropractor also may administer a more robust treatment, including a local high-velocity thrust, to move a joint. By reducing or eliminating a source of irritation to the spinal nerves, the body will be allowed to operate more efficiently and comfortably.

Chiropractic science was pioneered by American anatomist Daniel Palmer in 1895. Since 1974, standards for chiropractic education have been established and monitored by the Council on Chiropractic Education. Today there exist sixteen chiropractic colleges in the U.S. offering a four-year program that heavily emphasizes anatomy and physiology, and it is the third largest health care profession in the western world after allopathic (conventional) medicine and dentistry.

## Shiatsu

Shiatsu, meaning in Japanese "pressure" (*atsu*), "with fingers" (*shi*), was developed at the beginning of the twentieth century and is derived from an ancient form of Japanese massage introduced from China in the sixth century A.D. As described above, all the body's major systems (circulatory, nervous, musculoskeletal, digestive, etc.) are sheathed in connective tissue. Since any movement generates a bioelectric signal, tensions are carried through the connective tissue network (the meridians). As with other manual therapies, touch is used to assess the flow and distribution of energy throughout the body. The therapist applies many different kinds of pressure along the body's meridians and other sensitive pressure points with the fingers, palms, elbows, and knees, which induces tiny electric currents. These signals help rearrange tissues, making them more conductive in order to remove blockages and to trigger the self-healing process. There is simultaneously an improvement in microcirculation and in the oxygenation of tissues, which helps flush out toxins and waste products. Shiatsu may also involve light, rhythmic movements, as well as gentle stretching and manipulation. Sessions usually take place on a futon or mattress placed on the floor and are performed through loose-fitting clothing.

Another version of the same process is *acupressure*, a noninvasive form of acupuncture where the body is stimulated to release endorphins (a group of amino acids produced by the pituitary gland), which, when released into the bloodstream, act upon the central nervous system to help suppress pain and produce a sense of calm.

Shiatsu is useful during and after pregnancy to tone the body's Qi (energy) and restore imbalances. In the postnatal period, it is very helpful in overcoming the baby blues and excessive tiredness, constipation, and lactation difficulties.

Full shiatsu training is three years long, and, as with all manual therapies, is best undertaken after formal training as a health practitioner.

## Reflexology

Reflexology is a sophisticated form of foot massage or manipulation in which the feet represent a map of the whole body. It evolved from Chinese medicine and is based on the theory that energy pathways link the feet and hands to the rest of the body. Thus the reflexology points in the feet act as nerve receptors for all the organs of the body.

An American physician, William Fitzgerald, observed that a patient's perception of pain could be affected by pressing elsewhere on the body. At the beginning of the twentieth century, he divided the body into ten longitudinal zones in order to treat disorders by working on areas of the hand or foot representing that zone. This was the beginning of modern reflexology in the U.S. In the 1930s, the massage therapist Eunice Ingham, who studied with Fitzgerald, was the first to use the "grip" technique, whereby the thumbs and forefingers move across the foot, covering its every point. By enervating the more than seven thousand nerves on the feet, reflexologists claim to reach every muscle system and organ in the body.

In reflexology, therapists do not aim to treat an illness but rather to stimulate the innate capacity of the body to rebalance itself towards optimal health. The compression massage that is often used also aids in eliminating the crystalline deposits of excess calcium and uric acid which accumulate under the skin when the body's metabolism is disrupted.

The therapist will examine the feet for swelling, discoloration, and dryness, all signs of a disorder in the corresponding zone of the body. As the area relating to the affected organ is being worked on, the patient may feel a pinpricking sensation (as if the therapist were sticking his or her nails into the foot). This is often the sign of an acute or current disorder.

Reflexology is also useful in stress relief and relaxation. In the post-natal period, new mothers have found it effective in alleviating constipation, perineal discomfort, excessive bleeding due to subinvolution (the uterus is not returning fast enough to its nonpregnant state), hemorrhoids, lactation problems, as well as depression and anxiety.

# I

# The First
# Few Days

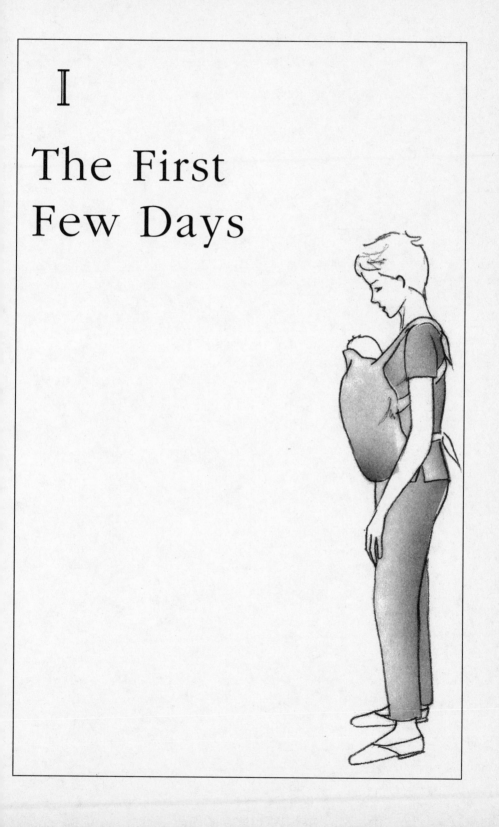

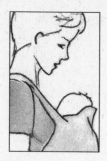

# 1

# A Great Physical Upheaval

In the hours after giving birth, most women feel a marvelous sense of well-being. This state of euphoria is caused by a rush of endorphins, the hormones that produce feelings of happiness and elation (the same ones that are stimulated by alcohol, drugs, and . . . chocolate). Some women may feel drowsy, the way one feels after sitting in the sun for several hours, or have an irresistible urge to sleep. Others may experience a burst of energy and excitement that makes them extremely receptive to the new baby.

If you have given birth vaginally, you will be kept under observation for about two hours in the delivery room, then taken to your room and put to bed. Your temperature, pulse, and blood pressure will be checked, as well as the amount of blood on your sanitary pad, and the location and firmness of the fundus (top of the uterus).

Although you may be resting, your body is already going back to work. Its next job is almost as demanding as the task it accomplished over the past nine months. During pregnancy, it provided all the components necessary for the gestation of a human being. During the delivery, it opened itself up and became supple to allow the baby's passage. Now, it must undertake a process of healing and closure in order to return to its pre-pregnancy proportions. One aspect will be the elimination of the excess tissue, water, blood, and other fluids produced over the previous nine months. The driving force behind this enormous undertaking is the hormonal revolution required to overturn the functions of pregnancy. As we shall see, the process may be a bit bumpy and various problems may arise. Fortunately, remedies exist for each one.

## The Hormonal Revolution

Throughout this book, we will refer frequently to hormones, the "links between the body and the mind" that play such an important part in controlling our emotions and many of the physical mechanisms in our bodies. Hormones (from the Greek word for "to encourage") are required to set in motion all vital functions. Their role is particularly important during pregnancy and the postnatal period. Medicine has not yet advanced enough to master hormonal changes. In fact, no linear cause-and-effect relationship has yet been found between the amount of a hormone secreted and the intensity of symptoms a woman feels. The way each of us reacts to a hormonal surge or dip depends on our physical and psychological health, and on our environment. Our reactions are therefore unpredictable, especially the first time we experience a major event such as childbirth.

### During Pregnancy

During pregnancy, the ovaries secrete large doses of hormones such as *estrogen*, which will stimulate the development of the uterus and breasts, increase the production of proteins needed for fetal growth, and cause the body's muscles and ligaments to become more supple. Another hormone secreted by the ovaries, *progesterone*, inhibits the contraction of the body's smooth muscles so that the uterus does not go into premature labor (other smooth muscles such as the intestines or the urinary tract also slow down, which explains why so many pregnant women are constipated or have urinary infections). The other major "production center" for pregnancy hormones is the placenta.

## After Delivery

With the expulsion of the placenta, the body suddenly stops producing these hormones. Within hours, their levels will plummet (estrogen levels, for example, drop by 90 percent!). For many women, the brutality of this drop is hard to take and contributes to emotional reactions such as "baby blues" and, in part, postnatal depression.

During pregnancy, the levels of the principal milk production hormone, *prolactin*, also multiplied by ten to twenty-fold. After delivery, prolactin levels drop, but still remain higher than normal for four to six weeks. If the mother is breastfeeding, she will experience prolactin peaks during this period. Afterwards, breastfeeding will function independently of this hormone.

*Oxytocin*, the hormone that stimulates uterine contractions, plays a very important role during childbirth and throughout the postnatal period. Oxytocin also is released when the brain recognizes that a baby is sucking on the breasts. This explains why women can feel their uterus contract while the baby is nursing (for some women, these nursing contractions are quite painful, for others, they are incredibly pleasurable, even close to the sensation of an orgasm).

Between the twenty-fifth and forty-fifth day after childbirth, estrogen is once again produced in sufficient quantity to initiate a menstrual cycle towards the thirty-fifth day after childbirth (nursing mothers may experience a much longer wait).

### A FEW WORDS OF ADVICE

Mothers who choose not to breast-feed should nevertheless wear a maternity bra for several days after giving birth, both day and night (until their milk supply dries up and their breasts are disengorged) as they probably will leak colostrum and milk. They should shower normally but try not to manipulate their breasts.

It is important to note that breast infections can also strike women who do not nurse but who still become engorged, or those who suddenly stop nursing while their breasts are still engorged. Fortunately, when treated in a timely manner, 99 percent of breast problems present a minimum risk of complication.

# The Reproductive System

The uterus can be compared to a hot-air balloon anchored by ligaments to the front, rear, and sides of the pelvis. Uterine fibers stretch to
some forty times their original size. The "balloon's" weight goes from
two ounces (about the size of a small pear) to more than two pounds
(the weight of a large watermelon). After delivery, it is faced with the
massive task of contraction and shrinking to recover its normal volume.
This is called involution. For nine months, the entire genital apparatus
is engorged with the blood that is required to nourish the fetus. Once
the baby is born, the body must dispose of all this excess blood.

## After Childbirth

The uterus shrinks to the size it was during the fifth month of pregnancy. Once the placenta is expelled, it contracts and appears like a little ball, hard to the touch when prodded through the abdominal wall
(this is why doctors and nurses will continually be poking your stomach in the days after childbirth). As soon as the uterus starts to soften,
the brain automatically knows to set off a contraction that will tighten
the uterine fibers and compress its blood vessels, in order to prevent
them from bleeding. During the first twelve hours after childbirth, these
after-pains can be as strong as labor contractions—though much less
painful. Gradually weaker contractions may continue for as long as a
week after childbirth.

## After Each Successive Birth

Even after just one pregnancy, the uterus will forever be slightly lower.
At each birth, a woman will have stronger and more frequent contractions since each baby will leave the uterus a little larger and less
toned—thus requiring a little harder work to recover its normal size.

Involution is rapid in the beginning (the uterus can no longer be
felt after about ten days and returns to its normal size in about fifteen
days). The process slows down during the third week and is not fully
complete until about two months after childbirth.

# The Recovery Process

The recovery process begins with the expulsion of the placenta a few minutes after the baby's birth. The postpartum contractions described above compress the blood vessels that fed the placenta. At the same time, an army of white blood cells arrives to restructure the uterine lining (*endometrium*) by digesting the topmost layer of blood-starved cells. This waste is sloughed off and discharged as *lochia* (postpartum bleeding similar to menstrual flow). The average amount of lochia expelled is about one pint, three-quarters of which flows out within the first four days.

The discharge will be heavy and bright red for the first four days as it contains mostly blood from the implantation site and cells from the topmost uterine layer, as well as small clots and bits of mucus. Toward the fifth day, the discharge will become pale pink. At this stage, it contains the white blood cells that have accomplished their cleaning task, old uterine tissue, and excess fluids. Starting around the tenth day, the lochia turns yellowish-pink to creamy-white, as it contains primarily white blood cells and uterine tissue. While the top layer of the uterus is being broken down and sloughed off, new cells are building up a fresh uterine lining below. Within about three weeks, the restructuring of the inner surface will be complete, except at the implantation site of the placenta. A different process takes place here, in order to avoid any scarring which could obstruct future pregnancies. Over a period of six weeks, the cells gradually regener-

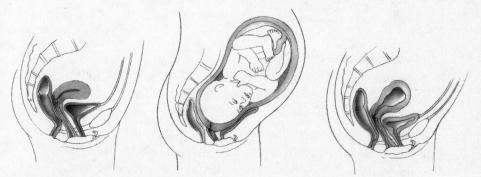

**The three sizes of the uterus**
*The position of the uro-genital organs before pregnancy, before delivery, and just after childbirth. Once the menstrual cycle resumes, the uterus is back to its pre-pregnancy size.*

# RECOVERING FROM CHILDBIRTH

## Homeopathy

As soon as possible after giving birth, a dose of Arnica 30CH will help overcome the physical and psychological shock to your body. This dose should be repeated every four hours during the twenty-four-hour period immediately following delivery.

The following remedies also are effective:

- One dose of China 9CH if you bled a lot during delivery.
- 3 granules Caulophyllum 5CH twice a day for three days to help the uterus return to its normal size.

If your bleeding is very heavy or prolonged:

- Arnica Montana 5CH (3 granules three times a day until the symptoms disappear) for heavy, bright red flows.
- China 5CH (in the same quantities) if the blood is dark.
- Kreosotum 5CH (3 granules in the evening) if the bleeding stings, itches, or causes a burning sensation (especially when you urinate).

## Minerals

- A tincture of copper, gold, and silver (1 teaspoon beneath the tongue every morning when you wake up) taken for three weeks will help lift your spirits and energy levels.
- Copper supplements, taken for three weeks, will help your body fight anemia by facilitating the absorption of iron in your body.

## Herbal Remedies

- Two essential oils help in toning the uterus: Palma Rosa and Cymbopogon martini. The latter also is useful in fighting infections and works as a general-purpose tonic. Take 3 drops on a sugar cube.
- Herbalists recommend drinking 2 to 3 cups daily for the first three to four days after childbirth of an infusion of Lady's Mantle combined with Raspberry leaf (a wonderful toner for the uterus) and Nettles. Then continue for four to six weeks with an infusion of Raspberry leaf and Nettle.

ate beneath the old tissue, healing the implantation site and completing the recovery process.

## Bleeding

It is normal to bleed for up to four to six weeks. Women sometimes tend to bleed more heavily after a cesarean section and lose blood during surgery. These women therefore run a greater risk of anemia. While the uterus is sloughing off its topmost layer, it is quite common to find blood clots on your sanitary pad, ranging in size from that of a penny to a cherry tomato. When the clot is particularly large, it may cause some pain as it is expelled from the body. This happens most often while nursing (as we have seen, the baby's sucking sends a signal to the brain to release oxytocin, which causes uterine contractions) or after a particularly strong after-pain. Never hesitate to show your sanitary pad to a nurse (someone should check your pad regularly in any case) if you feel that something abnormal is occurring. If the uterus is very distended (due to a large baby, twins, excess amniotic fluid, or repeated pregnancies that may have overstretched the uterine muscles), a new mother can bleed very heavily—without it being considered a real hemorrhage. Heavy bleeding can also result if there were placental insertion problems during the pregnancy (*placenta praevia*), or if there are uterine fibroids or certain other abnormalities present. In these cases, the doctor can administer oxytocin to help the uterine muscles contract so that new mother will not lose great amounts of blood and suffer from anemia or intense fatigue.

How long does heavy bleeding last? Generally not longer than four days, or a week at most. But it is normal to soak five or six special "extra-absorbent" sanitary pads in the first twenty-four hours (never use tampons until after your postnatal check-up).

Even though maternity wards provide sanitary dressings that are longer and more absorbent than those found in drugstores, you may want to use two pads, one over the other. While you are lying down, blood tends to accumulate and coagulate in the vagina and can cause an unpleasant gush when you get up. It is handy to have an extra sanitary napkin close at hand, which you can add to your dressing, so that you can walk to the bathroom without leaving an embarrassing trail. For the first week after childbirth, plan to use disposable underwear or panties that you won't mind throwing away. You may also want to place a disposable "incontinence sheet" over your bottom sheet (available in most drugstores), as is done in many hospitals.

# A FEW USEFUL ADDITIONS TO
# YOUR HOSPITAL SUITCASE

• A few plastic bags or large cosmetic cases in which to keep your sanitary pads and nursing pads clean and private. Nurses tend to show up with these items in large open boxes.

• Some moist antibacterial towelettes to wipe toilet seats, especially if you are sharing a bathroom. Even if the bathroom is cleaned regularly, you are surrounded by women who are losing blood—and blood is an ideal environment for germs.

• Your own pillow. The smell and texture will be comforting to you. Hospital pillows are often covered with a plastic liner.

• Three nursing bras. Mothers-to-be are often advised to buy only one nursing bra before giving birth, because they do not know what size they will be when they begin nursing. But it is advisable to have three bras (a size larger than the one worn at the end of pregnancy) ready in the first days when leaks are almost inevitable.

• Nightgowns or nightshirts that are made of sturdy fabric (preferably cotton) and open in the front. You probably will be sweating a lot, leaking milk, and burping a newborn who may spit up frequently. Large T-shirts are not practical if you want to nurse outside of bed, because nothing will cover up your lower body. T-shirts also have the annoying habit of falling onto the baby's face. Later, when you are more practiced at nursing, the type of clothing you wear will matter less. Some women prefer pajamas, but be careful about the size, as your belly will still be large: the top may fit, but the bottom might still be too small. If you use the hospital gown or "Johnny," put it on backward with the opening in the front.

• A dressing gown or bathrobe that closes well (better yet, that buttons), so as not to be uncovered while you are nursing outside your bed or walking the halls and visiting the nursery.

• A pair of slippers that are looser or larger than your normal size, because your feet will be swollen with the water retention that follows childbirth.

- Your favorite beauty supplies (including a mineral water mister), a hypoal-lergenic deodorant, a good moisturizer, and a little makeup for all the photographs. Between the sweating, the bleeding, and the milk leaks, you may not feel very eager to see visitors (women who deliver by cesarean section may not be able to shower for several days). And don't forget lip balm, because lips get very dry and chapped during labor when you breathe primarily through your mouth.

- The homeopathic remedies, herbal teas, and essential oils recommended in this book.

- A dress or a shirt that buttons in the front (something from your mater-nity wardrobe or two sizes larger than your pre-pregnancy size) that you can wear to leave the hospital. Chances are high you'll have to nurse the baby just when you're being discharged, especially if the formalities take a long time.

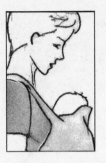

2

# Caring for the Genital Organs

## The Uterus

As described in the previous chapter, the contractions or "after-pains" that occur after delivery are necessary to compress the uterine blood vessels so as to prevent hemorrhaging. They usually begin during the first twenty-four hours after delivery and normally last between one and four days, or up to a week in some rare cases (if they persist longer than a week, it could be the sign of a uterine infection requiring immediate medical attention). During the first two days, after-pains can be so strong that they take your breath away.

### Coping with After-pains

Anticipate the spasms. Since after-pains often occur while breast-feeding, make certain that you are comfortably seated in a calm environment. Try a few breathing exercises (see pages 228–229) to relax before nursing.

Empty your bladder frequently, especially before nursing. As the

**Lying on your stomach helps ease after-pains**
*Many women find it comfortable to place small pillows under their head, hips, and ankles. Pillows can also be positioned under the rib cage to relieve pressure on the breasts. This is also a good way to alleviate congestion in the pelvic floor.*

bladder fills, it pushes back the uterus, which prevents it from contracting properly. The uterus will continue attempting to contract, which will cause prolonged, though ineffective, after-pains. It is therefore advisable to urinate frequently, especially the second and third day.

Lie on your stomach with a pillow under your abdomen, to put pressure on the uterus. If your breasts are squashed, elevate the top part of your chest with another pillow in order to create a hollow for the breasts (see diagram).

Do breathing and relaxation exercises (see pages 228–229).

Sleep on your side or on your stomach, with a pillow pressed against the uterus. This hurts for a few minutes in the beginning, but as soon as the uterus hardens it will feel better. It is also possible to nurse in this position with the baby properly propped among cushions.

If you are having a spasm, stop whatever you are doing. Close your eyes and concentrate on your abdominal muscles so that they relax as much as possible. With one hand, press on the pubic bone. Cross your legs. Bend forward. With the palm of your other hand, press on the uterus, which you will feel through the lower part of your belly. Gently jiggle your stomach if it is not too painful. Breathe deeply.

## Massaging the Uterus

External massages are useful to assist the uterus in its shrinking process and to soothe after-pains. This exercise also is useful just before nursing. The harder the uterus, the less it will contract under the surge of oxytocin released by the baby's sucking (but this massage is just as important if you are not breast-feeding).

# AFTER PAINS

## Homeopathy

- 4 granules Cuprum 5C (copper) in the morning, 4 granules Cimifuga 5C at noon, 4 granules Cuprum 5C before dinner, and 4 granules Cimifuga 5C before bed. Or else, 3 granules Silicea 5C every two hours. Normally, you should notice some easing of the pain after sixteen hours, and the pain should disappear after twenty-four hours.

In addition, you may wish to consider the following:

- If general exhaustion and muscular weakness accompany the pains: Caulophyllum, 5C three times a day.
- If the pains make you feel very hot: Pulsatilla 5C three times a day.
- If the pains feel like a heaviness or if you find yourself bearing down as if your uterus were going to fall out: Sepia 5C three times a day.
- If you have excessive bleeding or are passing clots and your pain girdles the pelvic area: Sabina 5C three times a day.
- If you had excessive bleeding during the birth and you are dehydrated: China 5C three times a day.
- If the painful after-pains occur while you are nursing: 4 granules Magnesia Phosphorica 5C just before nursing.
- If you suffer from abrupt abdominal pains that send pain throughout the lower belly and thighs: Viburnum Opulus 5C.
- If the pain feels like small contractions that are hard to locate, with a pulling sensation in the lower belly: Caulophyllum 5CH.

To help the uterus return to its normal size:

- If the uterus is swollen and hard: Aurum Nuriaticum Natronatum 5CH.
- If the uterus feels bloated with retained fluids and causes great pain: Lilium Tigrinum 5CH.
- If you feel sore in the abdominal or uterine areas: Bellis Perennis 5CH.

## Herbal Remedies

Brew an herbal tea consisting of Achillea or Millefolium (yarrow) (30 grams per quart of water), using just the blossoms or the whole plant without its roots. Drink 3 cups three times a day. These plants have an antispasmodic effect.

---

**Aromatherapy**

Essential oil of Tarragon (Artemisia Dracunculus) is a remarkable antispasmodic, which also has beneficial effects on the gastro-intestinal system.

---

Feel the uterus by prodding your belly between the navel and the pubic bone. If you can't feel it, move upwards a bit towards your chest, pressing quite hard. A nurse can also guide you.

+ Rub the area in small circles, about two inches around the navel.
+ The uterus should react by contracting: you may feel a small, hard ball developing, about the size of a grapefruit.
+ Try to massage yourself every four hours, especially just before nursing, so as to minimize the contractions.
+ Beware: You may notice that your bleeding increases following a massage. This is the uterus regenerating itself. The contraction stimulated by the massage will cause the uterus to work harder at sloughing off its spent lining. You may want to wear an extra sanitary napkin, or have one on hand for a fresh change.

If the after-pains are severe, you may be offered nonsteroidal antinflammatories such as ibuprofen (Advil or other) or acetaminophen (Tylenol). Occasionally, you may need stronger pain medication such as Percodan or Tylenol with codeine. These should be taken between feedings to minimize the amount transferred to the baby.

## The Birth Canal

For the first twenty-four hours following a vaginal delivery, the whole genital area will feel tender but rather numb. Then, as sensation returns, the dull ache will be replaced by the soreness associated with bruising. The intensity of any pain will depend on how much the passages have been dilated by the delivery, and whether any medical intervention was required (episiotomy, forceps, etc.).

The cervix will remain a little dilated for up to a week. Then it will thicken, shrink, and return to its initial shape. By looking at the cervix, a medical practitioner can tell if a woman has given birth vaginally, as it will appear like a line, whereas before the cervix resembled a small hole at the end of a tube. The cervix sometimes tears slightly, but in almost all cases, the wound will heal by itself.

The vagina is swollen and smooth for a day or two. During the following three or four weeks, it will shrink and return almost to its original dimensions. The vaginal walls, pelvic muscles, and ligaments will remain more supple for two to three months.

The external genitalia also changes: both the large and small lips double in size, the vulva and the anus have slackened (few women realize that stools and urine also were ejected during the expulsion of the baby).

Even if the delivery occurred smoothly, without an episiotomy, the pressure of the baby's head on the perineum and the distension of the vagina (it opens more than four inches) will inevitably cause some bruising and irritation. The genital area will therefore be very sensitive during the week that follows delivery.

## Possible Complications

**Hematomas** (swelling or collection of blood beneath the skin): This can occur after an episiotomy or repair of a laceration. Very rarely, a rupture in the deeper blood vessels creates a painful pocket of blood or a clot in the blood vessel (*thrombus*). Hematomas must be watched because they can become infected. More frequently, the vessels around the anus break and small clots of blood form beneath the skin, especially if you push too hard during bowel movements.

**Tears:** Despite the perineum's extraordinary capacity to distend, the skin and even the muscles frequently tear (30 to 60 percent of women who do not have an episiotomy tear during their first delivery).

A small tear in the outer genitalia or vaginal lining is sewn up in several minutes and complications are rare. It will scar in about twenty-four hours. A more serious situation occurs when there is a vertical tear through muscles and skin. If it is stitched correctly (generally in less than half an hour), complications are rare. The perineum is well irrigated by blood vessels, which bring the necessary nutrients to enable speedy healing. Sometimes, the tear reaches the external fibers of the anal sphincter wall (which is situated nearest the vagina), but the anal lining stays intact.

When modern delivery practices are applied correctly, one rarely hears of the major tears into the rectum that plagued women in the past. If this does happen, it must be surgically stitched but it generally heals easily.

It is also possible, but rare, that the perineum's muscles can tear underneath the surface of the skin, while the skin stays intact. This may go unnoticed at the time of delivery but the pain in the days following delivery will be intense. In such cases, the doctor or midwife will prescribe bed rest so that the muscles can repair themselves rapidly.

Sometimes, the vaginal lips will tear. This wound is painful for two to four days, and will burn if splashed with urine. It will heal on its own.

How long does the irritation last? If the perineum stays intact, or has only had a small tear, the irritation caused by bruising and stretching will disappear in fewer than ten days. But most women feel some pain from a larger tear, an episiotomy, or a difficult delivery for two to three weeks after delivery, and the pelvic region will remain sensitive for much longer (especially during sexual intercourse).

## After an Episiotomy

This is an incision (either lateral or midline) of the lower perineum muscles of the vulva made as a preventive measure to avoid tearing of the perineum and to facilitate the baby's expulsion. It is also said to protect the mother from urinary incontinence and, in the long term, from a prolapse (falling organs).

When an episiotomy is not performed, the perineum tears about half the time during a first delivery. Except in very serious cases, the skin heals naturally, but the muscles can remain fragile. Many obstetricians and midwives claim that it is easier to stitch tissue that was cut neatly by scissors than to sew torn tissue. They prefer to make an incision ahead of time and cut the muscle, rather than risk a jagged tear that they find more difficult to repair.

Since babies tend to be larger these days (thanks to better prenatal nutrition and to progress in obstetrics), episiotomies are increasingly common and the cut often is also longer. Without wanting to

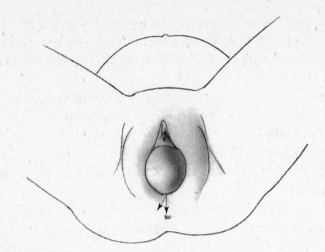

**The episiotomy**
*Depending on the practitioner, the incision will be either diagonal or vertical.*

enter the current debate on episiotomies, we simply wish to point out
that an episiotomy is not the only means available to protect the birth
canal:

+ The woman's position during delivery, the way she pushes,
  and her efforts to get back into shape after childbirth have just
  as much influence in avoiding future urinary incontinence or
  prolapsed organs as an episiotomy.
+ An episiotomy will not prevent the baby's head from crushing
  the urethra against the pubic bone, causing temporary urinary
  problems.
+ An episiotomy does not always avoid a complete rupture of
  the perineum into the rectum (especially if the baby has a big
  head, if the head is pointing in the wrong direction, or if the
  use of forceps is required).
+ Earlier arguments in favor of episiotomies were valid when
  there was no choice but to let tissues tear and heal by themselves. When scar tissue is torn repeatedly, it will no longer
  heal properly. Today, women are in better physical condition
  and are better prepared for delivery. A growing number of
  doctors and midwives prefer to use the episiotomy only when

## A PRACTICE THAT VARIES FROM COUNTRY TO COUNTRY

The use of episiotomy varies from country to country, depending on the opinions of the medical community. In the United States, it is used for 90 percent of women having their first child, and 62 percent of all women. In Spain, Italy, and Austria, it is practiced on 90 percent of women. On the other side of the spectrum, in the Netherlands, where midwives manage most deliveries from start to finish, the episiotomy rate is 10 percent. In Great Britain, the practice is used in 30 percent of births attended by midwives, and 90 percent of those attended by a doctor.

Techniques also differ from one country to another. For example, in Europe and Australia, most episiotomies are cut in a mediolateral direction so as to avoid tears in the rectum. In the United States and Canada, midline incisions in the center of the perineum are considered less traumatic because there are fewer nerves and blood vessels in the middle of the muscle.

the baby must come out quickly or if instruments such as forceps or a vacuum extractor are necessary.

## How the Episiotomy Is Performed

When the baby's head presses against the perineum, compressing the blood vessels (which minimizes the bleeding), the doctor or midwife inserts a finger between the head and the edge of the vagina and cuts a clean, straight line (most often towards the right, as most doctors are right-handed).

## Stitching the Episiotomy

Once the baby is born and the delivery over, the episiotomy is sewn layer by layer (the vaginal wall and then the perineal muscle) with a quick-absorbing vicryl thread. The skin is then usually sewn with a self-absorbing thread. If you notice a tiny piece of white or colored thread on your sanitary napkin, it is probably part of a stitch that was half-absorbed by your body.

# HEALING
# THE VAGINAL AREA

### Herbal Remedies

Dab the vulva with a tincture of Witch Hazel, Calendula, or with a mixture of water and medicinal clay. You can also use a compress soaked in lavender or chamomile oil, which helps reduce inflammation (use a very diluted mixture which will not sting when applied to an irritated area).

A warm decoction of Oak Bark, Comfrey Bark, Marigold and Lavender flowers also can be used on compresses. If however there is deeper damage or the risk of an infection, add 1 tablespoon of Slippery Elm and Golden Seal powders in equal quantities to the decoction before making a compress. Soak the perineum for twenty minutes twice a day (once a day if you have stitches). Doing pelvic floor exercises while applying the compress will help draw the healing fluid into the vagina.

When the area is simply abraded but the skin has not been cut or torn, apply a few drops of Italian Everlasting (Helichrysum Italicum) essential oil in a base oil directly to the vulva.

Some women find that soaking sanitary pads in one of these solutions and then freezing them is a nicer alternative than the proverbial bag of frozen peas.

If you have not had an episiotomy, massaging the area with arnica or calendula cream may help alleviate discomfort.

Take a warm sitz bath containing a few drops of calendula tincture.

The following lotion can be applied four times a day: 1 milliliter of essential oil of Chamomile in 30 milliliters of an equal mixture of Calendula and Millepertuis oils. To strengthen the mucous membranes, drink infusions of Marigold, Wild Indigo, Golden Rod, Ground Ivy, and Plantain. Another good infusion for the recovery of the genital area is made with Nettle, Motherwort, Lemon Balm, Hawthorn Berry (leaf and flower), and Fennel. Also remember to eat zinc-rich foods such as ginger, parsley, potatoes, garlic, turnips, carrots, rye, oats, and buckwheat.

### Homeopathy

- Staphysagria 7CH: 2 granules, morning and evening, for three or four days to accelerate the healing process throughout the genital area.
- Apis 9CH: 3 granules twice a day for three or four days to alleviate bruising and congestion.

## Caring for the Genital Area

### If You Did Not Have an Episiotomy

In all cases, the genital area must be carefully cleaned and cared for.

Rinse the genital area with a stream of warm water from the perineal cleansing bottle ("peri" bottle) supplied by the hospital after every trip to the bathroom.

Remove every trace of urine and dried blood after urinating with warm water in a peri bottle and dry with cotton balls or gauze.

To prevent the blood that accumulates in your sanitary pad from sticking to your skin, pour a few drops of witch hazel lotion (available in most pharmacies) onto the sanitary pad.

## Coping with Episiotomy Pain

As it is located in a part of the body that is almost always moist, the episiotomy scar is quite vulnerable to infection. Furthermore, the blood on your sanitary pad provides the perfect environment for bacteria to multiply. In most maternity wards, a nurse will inspect and clean your episiotomy scar over a bedpan once or twice after you deliver. As soon as you feel up to it, you can do this yourself by running warm water over your perineum in the shower (if you have a removable showerhead) or with cupfuls of warm water while standing over the toilet or bathtub. The soothing effect is immediate.

+ Wash your hands, especially in the hospital, where germs are more numerous than at home.
+ Always dry yourself from the front towards the back with a sterile compress (don't use a washcloth or sponge as long as the wound has not healed). When you are changing your sanitary pad, try to remove it by pulling it out towards the back.
+ Change sanitary napkins every four to six hours, or, better yet, every time you urinate.
+ Wash the area every time you go to the bathroom by running water over it as described above.
+ If you find that urine burns your scar every time you go to the bathroom, try slowly pouring cold water over the perineum as you urinate.

◆ Many pregnancy books recommend a hair dryer for drying the episiotomy scar, but we feel that this technique has huge drawbacks. It tends to dry out the perineum, dilate the blood vessels, and blow dust and bacteria right onto the open wound. (Some hospitals even forbid hair dryers). If you absolutely must use a hair dryer, choose one that has a cold air setting. Keep it six inches from the wound, and do not use it for more than 3 minutes at a time.

## Easing Episiotomy Pain

The healing process is usually painful, but to varying degrees of time and intensity. You may feel sore for twenty-four hours, for several days, or even for a few weeks.

During the first days, the perineum tissues will be swollen. As they swell, the skin pulls on the stitches. If the stitches are made of nylon, they will pull the most during the first few days, but will have relaxed by the fifth or sixth day. It is essential however that the tissues under the skin knit back together without too much tension. The skin itself generally forms its own scar within twenty-four hours.

For the majority of women, the scar is sore for about five days.

It can happen—although rarely—that intense pain will last for more than five days. If so, you should have the area checked to ensure that a hematoma (pocket of blood) has not formed which could become infected, and that the episiotomy scar itself has not become infected.

The pain should have almost entirely disappeared by the end of two weeks. If it persists, consult your doctor or midwife. If the problem is a badly absorbed stitch or a small infection, it can be treated and remedied quickly.

For some women, though, an irritating soreness will hamper sexual activity for as many as six months or more. "Did they sew me up properly?" "Will I be the way I was before?" are the questions most frequently asked by new mothers. These questions are especially loaded with sexual significance for first-time mothers, who don't dare ask directly, "Will I still be desirable?"

Hot or cold? Specialists do not agree on whether to use heat or cold to ease episiotomy pain. Practitioners of Chinese medicine say that pain is stagnant energy, and that heat makes this energy circulate. Others say that swelling causes the pain and that cold is required to ease swelling.

## Using Cold to Soothe the Wound

Ask the nurses if you can keep a mist bottle of mineral water in the maternity ward's refrigerator and use it to spray the perineum after you urinate (this will be easy to do at home).

+ Add a few ice cubes to a pitcher of water that you pour over the perineum. (If the hospital doesn't have a freezer, have someone bring you ice cubes in a thermos).
+ Fill a latex glove (disposable examination glove) with water and ask the nurses to put it in the freezer (this is more comfortable than filling a latex glove with ice cubes). Once frozen, place it on your perineum over the sanitary napkin.

## Using Heat to Soothe the Wound

Pour a pitcher of warm water or hold a hand-held shower head between your legs and spray the area with warm water.

Some specialists recommend using cold first, then heat. Use cold for the first twenty-four hours to reduce the swelling, and then use heat to sooth the soreness, improve the blood circulation, and encourage the healing process. If you also have hemorrhoids (it is very common to have both at the same time, and it is easy to confuse the source of pain), you probably will be tempted to use the cold remedies indicated for a little longer.

Some practitioners recommend sitting as much as possible with your legs crossed (Indian style), leaning slightly forward, with a pillow under the edge of your buttocks. Or else, sitting with one leg crossed in front of you, and the other bent behind you. This way, the body's weight is not resting on the perineum, but rather on the bony part of your bottom (the *ischium*).

## Exercise

To soothe the pain of an episiotomy, get on all fours on your bed, with a large pillow in front of you.

+ Place your hands under the pillow.
+ Slowly lower your elbows to the mattress, and let your head and chest rest on the pillow.

# EPISIOTOMY PAIN

### Classical Medication

Most maternity wards offer acetaminophen (Tylenol) and nonsteroidal anti-inflammatories (NSAIDs). It is not necessarily bad to use them while breast-feeding, but they should be taken just after nursing, so that their effect can wear off before the baby feeds again.

### Homeopathy

Take Arnica Montana 9C (for pain and postoperative shock) and Sta-physagria 9C (for healing the scar) every two hours for the first two days and then three times a day. The pain should disappear within three days.

- To ease swelling caused by bruising, take 3 granules of Apis 9C twice a day for three or four days.

### Herbal Remedies

The remedies are the same as those listed for healing the vaginal area (compresses of witch hazel or of the lotion described on page 36 on the perineum for 20 minutes). Be careful not use anything that might irritate or infect the wound. Above all, do not overuse creams or compresses (no more than every third time you clean the area), so as not to dry out the scar.

### Aromatherapy

Aromatherapy is particularly suited to healing wounds caused by abrasion and bruising. The following mixtures may be applied locally:

- Essential oil of Lavandin Abrial (1 drop) and essential oil of Ciste (1 drop) in a base oil.

- Essential oil of Musk Rose in a base oil.

- Essential oil of Italian Everlasting (Helichrysum Italicum) in a base oil. This remedy is remarkably efficient. It can also be taken orally if you are not breast-feeding.

- Essential oil of Wood Rose in a base oil.

◆ Bring your knees slightly forward so that your back is rounded and "comfortable." Your buttocks will be in the air.

◆ Stay in this position for 5 to 10 seconds. Try to relax as much as possible. (In the beginning, you may feel that your blood is rushing toward your head.)

◆ To return to an upright position, push up on your hands until your arms are fully stretched. Unroll your back, one vertebra at a time, until you are back up on your knees.

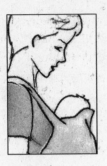

# 3

# Your Bodily Functions After Childbirth

G iven the upheaval that your organs have experienced during pregnancy and childbirth, they need a bit of time to recover their normal functions.

## Urination

After giving birth, it is extremely important not to let the bladder remain full for any length of time. Once the fetus is gone, the bladder suddenly has more room to expand. But it has lost tone (under the influence of pregnancy hormones) it can easily become overly distended. Furthermore, a full bladder pushes the uterus upwards and can prevent it from contracting, which in turn increases the risk of hemorrhage. This is why it is essential to empty the bladder within six hours after delivery. The nurse or midwife can help you.

Many women do not feel the need to urinate after giving birth. The urethra has been rubbed sore by the pressure caused by the baby's passage, and the sphincter may still be numb under the influence of the epidural anesthetic.

If the first attempt at urination is painful, it is normal to fear urinating again. Psychological factors can also cause urine retention: if you are still assigned to your bed, you will have to urinate in a bedpan. The lack of intimacy of a hospital room, the embarrassment of having to urinate in front of someone, and the discomfort of the bedpan make urinating difficult. The nurse can help by pressing gently on your bladder. If you still can't urinate, she will use a catheter.

Fortunately, urine-retention problems never last more than twenty-four hours. Be aware that blockage one day can be followed by frequent urination the next day, as the body begins to eliminate its excess liquids.

## A Few Tips to Help Induce Urination

In bed:

+ If you are sharing a room, ask the nurse to draw the curtain between the two beds.
+ Ask that the bedpan be warmed.
+ Sit on the bedpan rather than lie down over it.
+ Ask the nurse to pour warm water on your perineum; this sensation often stimulates urination.

### A FEW POINTERS ABOUT HYGIENE

It is well known that hospitals are germ repositories. On top of that, in a maternity ward, all the patients are bleeding profusely. A woman who has just given birth is particularly susceptible to infection in the genital area. Yet it is difficult not to "sit down" on the toilet when you are in pain or constipated or feeling very tired. In selecting a hospital or birth center you should ask if you will have a private bath. Many if not most maternity units in the U.S. now provide this amenity.

• Use antibacterial towelettes to wipe the toilet seat, especially if there are several people sharing the bathroom.
• Ask visitors not to use the toilets reserved for new mothers.
• Carry your sanitary napkins in a clean plastic bag that closes well.

In the bathroom:

+ Run the tap (the sound of running water can be suggestive).
+ Stand under a running shower.
+ Dip your fingers in hot water.
+ Press lightly on your bladder.
+ Pour a pitcher of warm water on your vulva.
+ Walk.
+ While urinating, lean forward so that the urine does not run over your episiotomy scar.

Be sure to clean your episiotomy scar each time you go to the bathroom.

## Fluid Retention

A pregnant woman's body holds more water than normal. The high level of estrogen increases the quantity of water between cells. In addition, the pressure of the uterus on the vena cava slows the drainage of these extracellular fluids. In the hours following delivery, many women note that their hands and feet have swollen.

Then, twenty-four hours after giving birth, the fall in estrogen levels and the disappearance of pressure on the vena cava allows the body's fluids to start returning to their pre-pregnancy levels. The change will happen rapidly—this is why, between the second and fifth day, you will need to urinate often. You will discharge almost 3 quarts of urine per day, instead of the habitual 1.5 quarts.

You also will perspire a lot, even excessively. This is called *diaphoresis*. Heavy nighttime sweating can last six to eight weeks and even up to a year for some women. Up to 10 percent of women have night sweats and hot flashes even after a month. It is normal and should not be prevented. But you will need to have some terrycloth towels that the nurses' aides can place between the plastic sheet and your bed sheets (or simply on top of the bed sheet) when they make up the bed. Also bring along extra nightgowns. If you want to, you may use some nonperfumed talcum powder, but be careful not to put powder on areas of your skin that will be in contact with the baby.

If your eyes are swollen and painful, do not hesitate to ask the nurses for icepacks (a bag of frozen peas will do just as well).

## Fluid Intake

For a long time, it was thought that new mothers should limit their intake of water so as to help their body to get rid of all the excess fluids accumulated during pregnancy. It was also thought that restricting fluids would prevent the breasts from becoming engorged with milk. Today, everyone recognizes that a new mother needs water to help the reproductive system clean itself, to reduce the acidity of her urine, and, above all, to produce milk. Do not limit your consumption of liquids! On the contrary, it is advisable to drink two quarts of water per day for the first days. Some hospitals even recommend adding sports drinks that contain electrolytes (such as Gatorade) so as to replenish the nutrients lost in childbirth.

## The Digestive Tract

During pregnancy, progesterone levels, some fifty times higher than normal, will not only prevent premature contractions of the uterus, but also the contractions of all the other smooth muscles of the body, such as the intestines. This slowing of the digestive system, coupled with the lack of exercise at the end of pregnancy, causes the constipation, bloating, acid reflux, and gas pains from which many pregnant women suffer. After childbirth, it takes several months for the digestive tract to return to its normal efficiency.

## Constipation: A Common Side Effect

Expect not to have a bowel movement for the first three days. Watch your diet in order to avoid constipating foods, because it is almost inevitable to be constipated during the week following delivery.

In the final stage of expulsion during delivery, the anus opens and the large intestine empties itself. Most women are not fed during labor and delivery (in cases of scheduled cesarean sections, the woman will have been fasting for eight hours before the procedure). As anyone who has been on a strict diet knows, it is easier to be constipated when you have nothing in your stomach. Anesthesia (whether epidural or general) also will slow down the intestinal functions. The tremendous pressure exerted on the rectum during expulsion leaves the tissues swollen. The swelling needs to ease in order to have a bowel movement. Some pain relievers (such as those with codeine) have a constipating effect. And weak abdominal muscles cannot help improve digestive functions. Finally, many women are afraid to have a bowel movement for fear of pulling their stitches or suffering hemorrhoids and irritating those already present (see pages 58 to 62).

## How to Soothe Constipation

+ Drink eight glasses (two quarts) of water per day.
+ Eat as few dairy products as possible during the first days. Avoid white bread, flour-based products, and chocolate.
+ Eat as many raw fruits and vegetables as possible (especially dried prunes and figs).
+ Walk.

The longer you wait, the harder and larger your stools will become. So, around the third day, summon your courage and go.

## Exercises

### Exercise 1
+ Stand up with your feet six inches apart, lean slightly forward, your hands on the front of your thighs. Inhale.
+ Exhale as far as possible (you should finish with a groan).
+ Holding your breath, suck your abdominal muscles inward, as though you wanted to pull them up against your spine.
+ Breathe in and relax your abdomen.

### Exercise 2
+ Repeat exercise 1, but this time, after you've exhaled, pull in and push out the abdominal muscles (as if to roll them in a sort of belly dance). Push outward, and then pull inward towards the spine. Try to do this three times.
+ Inhale and relax your abdomen.

### Exercise 3

+ Standing, press on the "energy point" on your lower belly (according to this Oriental concept, this energy point stimulates the intestines and relieves gas and constipation). To find it, put one hand on your stomach, with your thumb on your navel. The spot where your little finger is resting is this energy center. Press on it for four seconds. Repeat this three times in the morning and three times again in the evening.

### Exercise 4

+ Exhale as far as you can. Pull your abdominal muscles towards the back, and then upwards.
+ Inhale and relax.

In the beginning, it is normal to feel almost nothing, because the abdominal muscles are weak. We all know how to push our stomachs out, but it is harder to suck them in! The hardest part is learning to pull the muscles upwards. Throughout the day, remember to squeeze your buttocks very tightly, and then relax them. Once you have recovered from pregnancy and childbirth, the third exercise alone should be enough to relieve constipation.

A few tips for easier bowel movements:

+ Lean forward, and do not push while you are holding your breath.
+ If possible, when you are seated, raise your knees by resting your feet on two telephone directories or two boxes.
+ Take a sanitary napkin, fold it in half, press it against your stitches and try to relax your perineum.
+ If bowel movements are not happening spontaneously, tighten your stomach while exhaling.
+ Don't stay too long on the toilet. It is safer to provoke a bowel movement with a suppository or an enema than to push too hard.

Another helpful exercise is to massage your belly making large circles around the navel in a clockwise direction, from the position of 7

# CONSTIPATION

## Homeopathy

- 3 granules Hamamelis Virginiana 5C three times a day.
- If you have pain from gas, accompanied by bloating, Raphanus 5C every two hours until the gas is gone, then three times a day until stools are normal.
- If you do not have gas, 3 granules Thebalcum 9C two or three times a day can prove very effective.
- If you have dry, hard stools or difficulty in passing even a soft stool, and the problem is worse in the afternoon: Alumina 5C three times a day.
- If you are straining to have a movement and it is worse in the mornings: Nux Vomica 5C three times a day.
- If you have incomplete bowel movements with flatulence: Lycopodium 5C three times a day.
- If the constipation is stubborn and lasts for days, leaving you feeling like you have a ball in your rectum: Sepia 5C three times a day.

## Herbal Remedies

- Regularly drinking a glass of water containing a few grams of flaxseed (Linum usitatissimum), or sprinkling flaxseeds on salads and yogurts can soothe constipation. Drink 40 to 50 drops of Fumaria Officinalis tincture in water in the morning before breakfast.
- Tarragon is an herb well known for relieving constipation. Cinnamon is an antiseptic and digestive aid.
- The following infusion may be helpful: Dandelion Root Fennel, Beetroot Fibre, and Pysilium Husk.

## Aromatherapy

- Massage the left side of the abdomen, in a clockwise direction, with a mixture of 10 drops essential oil of Marjoram, 10 drops essential oil of Rosemary, 5 drops essential oil of Patchouli, and 5 drops essential oil of Fennel, diluted in 50 milliliters Sweet Almond oil.
- A combination of essential oils of Mandarin, Orange, Bergamot, Lime, and Grapefruit massaged over the belly in a clockwise direction also may be helpful.
- Make sure that you are getting enough vitamin C (1,000 mg a day).

o'clock to 5 o'clock. (It is important to rub in the clockwise direction, because that is the direction in which your intestines are laid out).

The nurse will probably offer you stool softeners (such as Colace), which will not affect the nursing baby. These should be taken two or three times per day. When you leave the hospital, continue taking them, but once a day. The recommendation is to continue the treatment until you have had two full weeks of clear improvement. Women who stop the treatment after two days of remission are sure to find themselves with the same problem again.

## Your First Exercises After Childbirth

### While in bed

- ✦ Curl your legs up on your stomach and press lightly on your knees while exhaling.
- ✦ Make small circles with your ankles.
- ✦ Write the letters of the alphabet (or the name of your baby!) with your feet.

## Walking

Most women have no trouble moving after childbirth. But some feel stiff and reluctant to move. Yet, it is extremely important to begin walking soon after the delivery, so as to avoid circulatory problems (see pages 57 and 90) and to encourage the elimination of excess fluids.

If the delivery was not complicated, you can generally get up out of bed as soon as the effects of the epidural wear off. The first time you get up, you will be assisted by a nurse (usually, the first time you get up is to go to the bathroom). The nurse should wait for you outside the bathroom door, and accompany you back to your bed. They usually do this automatically, but it doesn't hurt to make sure with a "Will you wait for me?" You may also get up to take a shower twelve hours after delivery.

It is important to walk, because walking helps drain the lower limbs, fights constipation, and prevents swelling and heaviness. If you are feeling very sore, here is a goal to work towards during your first few days: start out walking five to ten minutes and increase the amount each day.

## A FEW WORDS OF ADVICE

During the first six weeks, try to spend more time lying down than standing up. Avoid standing still for long stretches of time. Ask for a chair while you watch the baby being bathed in the nursery. (And do not forget to take your inflatable ring with you!) Remember that a few short walks are better than one long stroll.

After you have been standing, lie down and raise your pelvis slightly with a pillow. When you want to sit up, do not rise straight up from a lying position. First, roll over onto your side, and then push yourself up with your arms.

Remember to contract your perineum muscles before getting up or sitting down.

## Breathing

The physical upheaval that takes place in a woman's body during and after childbirth temporarily affects her respiratory ability. During the first week, her respiratory efficiency falls by 10 percent. This resulting excess of carbon dioxide in her system and lack of oxygen in the blood will accentuate fatigue.

On the first day, you will probably have just enough energy to take a few steps. But even without walking, you can still practice breathing exercises that are extremely beneficial. Breathing is important for:

- ✦ Relaxing.
- ✦ Controlling pain.
- ✦ Filling the emptiness in your stomach.
- ✦ Cleaning the body.
- ✦ Nursing: midwives have noticed that women who have trouble breast-feeding are tense because they are breathing poorly.

## Exercises

- ✦ Sitting as comfortably as you can in bed, with your eyes closed, concentrate on your body. Inhaling and exhaling, let the air run through you. Start with your feet and work towards your head. Associate every part of your body with a color.

This will help to "waken" a specific point in your body, and then to release it and oxygenate it.

◆ Lying on your bed, legs slightly apart, arms spread open and palms facing upwards, "rock" your pelvis from left to right in a pendulum swing. Yawn, then rock your ribs, then your chest, and finally your head. This exercise is an excellent way to make tension disappear from your body.

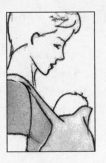

4

# Coping with the Side Effects of Childbirth

Most women have trouble sleeping through the night in their last weeks of pregnancy. They then often give birth in the middle of the night, may struggle through a long delivery, feel the intense excitement of the first hours of the baby's life, then get little sleep in the hospital—little wonder that many new mothers feel exhausted. A number of physical problems may also surface in the days after childbirth.

## The Common Side Effects of Childbirth

The first is **low energy** due to the body's sudden sensitivity to insulin (the hormone that regulates how our cells use sugar). During pregnancy, a woman is less sensitive than usual to the insulin level in her blood. But after delivery, a new mother becomes much more sensitive to insulin, as if she were on a strict diet. This may lead to a fatigue comparable to that of someone suffering from hypoglycemia.

The second is **weakness due to anemia**, which is caused by

## MASSAGE FOR CALMING SHIVERS AND TREMBLING

Place your hands on each side of your head, with your fingers on your forehead, and your thumbs on your temples. Slide your fingers forwards and backwards to find the point where your forehead is slightly more curved outwards. Let your head fall into your hands, pressing slightly with your fingers. Breathe slowly and feel a new sense of calm.

bleeding and slowed circulation (see page 57). Many women are anemic by the end of their pregnancy, while others become anemic *after* childbirth. For this reason, it is essential to keep taking your iron supplements (see also nutritional advice on page 136).

**Digestive difficulties, nausea or vomiting** linked to the anesthesia (epidural and especially general anesthesia), to the postoperative recovery from a cesarean section, to the morphine received after surgery, and to certain medicines are common. If morphine is administered intravenously, the doctor may also add a medicine to reduce nausea.

**Shivers and trembling** are commonplace and may last several days. They are due to the loss of heat in the body: the baby, placenta, and amniotic fluid, which together weighed about ten pounds at a constant temperature of 97°F. are no longer there. Another contributing factor may the posttraumatic shock of giving birth. There is little you can do other than ask for more blankets and try to relax (see page 228 for breathing exercises as well as the massages described below). The medical team should verify that these shivers and trembling are not caused by fever or by hypothermia, two signs of infection.

**Fever**. Towards the second day, some women develop a slight fever (100°F. or less), often just before their milk comes in. This should not last more than twenty-four hours. If you do get a fever, drink two or three quarts of water per day, and avoid aspirin, which thins the blood and may cause you to bleed more heavily. Instead, use acetaminophen (Tylenol), which is also effective in reducing fever. However, a fever higher than 100°F. is an alarm signal (see page 84).

**Headaches** may also occur after childbirth, and are essentially due to fatigue and tension. Relaxation exercises (see page 228, "Breathing")

---

## ACHES AND CRAMPS AFTER CHILDBIRTH

### Homeopathy

- If your legs and spine are sore (and if you feel cold, sleepy during the day, or have trouble urinating): 3 granules Causticum 5C in the morning.
- If the back pain spreads to your kidneys: 3 granules Nux Vomica 5C in the morning.
- If the pain radiates around your hips: 3 granules Silicea 5C in the morning.

### Aromatherapy

- Massage the sore area with an essential oil mixture of 50 percent Lavender and 50 percent Orange in a base oil. This will work as a relaxant and also help to fight stress (see also pages 226 to 229).

---

and Tylenol can soothe benign headaches. More rarely, a headache is the result of an epidural (see page 64). Headaches can also be caused by dehydration, so be sure you drink enough to replace the fluids lost during labor and delivery.

**Aches and cramps.** Some women complain about feeling sore all over, especially in their shoulders. When women deliver on their backs with their feet in gynecological stirrups, they often pull on the stirrups while pushing the baby out. Another very common reaction is to tighten your shoulders at every contraction. After delivery, some women also have sore arms and wrists (which can't be blamed on writing too many thank-you notes . . . yet). Your legs may also feel very tired, as though you had walked for miles. Aches and pains in the legs probably are due to having your legs bent back in stirrups for an extended period. After a cesarean, a pain under the ribs will come from the pocket of air that accumulates in the abdominal cavity during surgery (see page 70).

Ask the maternity ward nurses for a hot-water bottle, heat pack, or ice pack, to apply on the part of your body that is sore (or ask one of your visitors to purchase it on their way to the hospital).

**Carpal Tunnel Syndrome,** tingling in the hands, affects women during pregnancy or after childbirth. It is due to the fact that the major nerve-carrying signal between the brain and hand becomes severely pinched when surrounding tissues are swollen from the fluids of pregnancy. The problem will eventually resolve itself but may take as long as a year. Another form of "aches and pains" caused by pregnancy and childbirth is known as "Thoracic Outlet Syndrome," which is the compression of the brachial plexus in the armpit or right in front of the shoulder. It is caused by the heaviness of the breasts and uterus pulling the body forward. It may continue throughout the postnatal period when women tend to bend over more than usual in caring for their baby.

## Self-massage to Obtain Relief

Find the energy point in your shoulder by placing your right hand on your left shoulder, with your fingers along your neck. Then slide your fingers down toward the top of your shoulder, where the muscle feels rounded and protrudes slightly. (If you are not sure that you've found the right point, put your fingers on your left nipple, then move them upwards in a straight line right up to your shoulder, and stop just behind the crest of the shoulder).

+ Once you have found the point, press gently but firmly, drawing small circles that make the skin slide over the bone. Breathe in and out in a relaxed fashion.
+ Vary the pressure: press for four seconds, release for four seconds, but without lifting your fingers from the skin. Exhale while pressing down, inhale while releasing.
+ Start on this pressure point, rubbing with a circular motion, then go up a notch on the neck, and massage in circles. Continue, moving upwards a notch each time until you reach the crest of the backbone muscles on either side of the neck. Continue massaging in small circles until you reach the base of your skull. End by following the hairline right up to your temples.

**Weight**. A woman generally loses ten pounds during delivery, and between four and five pounds during the next few days. The other pounds will fall away gradually during the following months (see page 300).

**Backaches**. Many midwives report that half of new mothers suffer from backaches after giving birth. There are many potential reasons for a backache:

+ Bad posture during pregnancy, which exaggerates the curve of the lower back.

+ Lying on your back for a long period of time during delivery, with your legs up in stirrups, while the muscles and ligaments are artificially relaxed by the epidural anesthesia.

+ Pushing too hard in an uncontrolled manner during delivery may throw the pelvis off balance. Since the position of the pelvis determines the body's alignment, this is an important but often undetected cause of back pain.

+ A large baby may dislocate his mother's coccyx (tailbone). In one out of every ten vaginal deliveries, the coccyx is displaced. The pain can be intense and debilitating because the proper alignment of the coccyx is necessary for the body to move freely. If this happens to you, ask for one of the physical therapists on staff to treat you while you are still in the hospital. Better yet, if you have an existing relationship with a manual therapist (chiropractor, osteopath, etc.), ask for a bedside consultation, either while you are still in the hospital or as soon as you return home. The coccyx will need to be realigned before you can begin any childbirth recovery exercises. As a preventative measure, before checking in to the hospital, it might be wise to ask about their policy on allowing a therapist to treat you in your room after delivery. Many hospitals offer this service, but only on request. Otherwise, you may need to ask

---

### BACKACHE

**Homeopathy**
• If you are feeling weak and tired with dragging pains in the middle and lower back (and feel better for sitting and for warmth on your back): Kali Carb.
• If the pain comes on quickly, often on the right side, and is quite intense, possible accompanied by abdominal pain: Belladonna.
• If the pain is intense, spasmodic, with a tense feeling in the abdominals (and feels better for sleep and warmth): Nux Vomica.
• All should be taken in 30CH initially, three times a day, and during a pain attack.

your doctor for permission to bring your own therapist in
from outside.

+ Sudden loss of weight and muscle tone at the end of pregnancy causes soreness in most women, because their entire
alignment is altered, and the body must become accustomed
to its new size and shape.

+ The point in the lower back at which the epidural catheter
was inserted can remain sore for several days.

## Exercise

Do this in bed. This exercise soothes sore backs, tones the abdominal
muscles, and stimulates the intestines so as to minimize constipation.

+ Lie on your back with legs bent, feet flat on the mattress, hip-
width apart.
+ Draw your knees back over your stomach.
+ Inhale while relaxing for a moment in this position.
+ Exhale, try to curl your tailbone upwards (support your lower
back on the mattress), which lifts your buttocks up.
+ Hold for three seconds.
+ Relax. Repeat a few times.

## Circulatory Problems

During pregnancy, the future mother's blood volume increases by two
to four pints (this represents a gain of 35 to 40 percent) in order to
nourish the fetus and irrigate the uterus. This increased blood flow dis-
tends the thin, flexible walls of a pregnant woman's veins, notably in
the genital area. This explains why some women suffer from painful
varicose veins in the vulval area during pregnancy (these disappear
within hours of childbirth). During delivery, small blood vessels can
rupture under the pressure of pushing, especially in the face and
around the eyes. Cheeks and the upper chest area sometimes bruise.
These blue marks will disappear within several days.

Three weeks after giving birth, the mother's blood volume returns
to its normal, pre-pregnancy levels. One third of the excess blood will
have been lost in delivery, another through postpartum bleeding, and

the last third will be absorbed into her body. When these excess blood cells die, they simply will not be replaced.

In the hours following delivery, the blood's capacity to coagulate increases dramatically, while blood circulation slows down. The veins, full of slower-moving blood, become more visible (turning either blue or purple), especially on the breasts. The increased coagulation rate and the slower circulation prevent the body from losing dangerous amounts of blood after delivery, and insure the proper healing at the point where the placenta attached itself to the uterine wall.

However, these changes in the body's circulatory mechanisms also mean that there is an increased risk of blood pooling in the veins and of *thrombosis* (formation of blood clots in the veins), with the additional risk of *phlebitis* (inflammation of the veins). It is therefore very important to monitor a new mother's legs for swollen veins. The veins could become inflamed and provoke blood clots if the mother stays in bed on her back for too long. This is why doctors advise new mothers to get out of bed as soon as possible and to walk the hallways. If the new mother is at great risk of a circulatory problem (possesses risk factors such as obesity, cardiac problems, and previous circulatory troubles), she may be given daily injections of anticoagulants.

Another negative consequence of the slowed blood flow is the appearance, or aggravation, of anemia. As we have stated previously, it is extremely important to continue your pregnancy iron supplements, even if late-pregnancy blood tests showed that you were not iron deficient (see pages 136 and 137).

## Hemorrhoids

After the enormous physical exertion involved in giving birth, more than a third of women experience a hemorrhoid eruption about twenty-four hours after delivery. These are in fact swollen veins located just under the membrane that lines the lowest part of the rectum and anus. In addition, small blood vessels in the area may rupture and blood clots become visible under the skin. Women who have had an episiotomy are especially at risk (but since the whole genital area is sore, it is hard for them to differentiate perineal pain from that of hemorrhoids). This pain can be intense, especially when seated on a hard surface or when having a bowel movement.

---

## CIRCULATORY PROBLEMS

### Homeopathy
- Pulsatilla 5C, taken three times a day, is excellent for toning veins and capillaries.
- If you have fragile blood vessels: Lachesis.
- If you have an injury or trauma to the veins due to childbirth: Hamamelis (also good when phlebitis threatens).

### Herbal Remedies
- Cumin helps improve circulation and also acts as an antiseptic, as does parsley, which is both a diuretic and a blood purifier.

---

Seventy percent of women get hemorrhoids at some point during pregnancy or after deliver. Thirty percent of them are still bothered by hemorrhoids one month after the baby's birth, and 11 percent still have a problem after six months.

Hemorrhoids are provoked by:

+ A mechanical problem: the uterus is compressing the blood vessels of the lower abdomen, causing swelling in the veins around the anus.
+ The increased estrogen levels of pregnancy make blood vessel walls more fragile.
+ Constipation affects many pregnant women, forcing them to push harder when they want to have a bowel movement. This pushing can rupture the weakened blood vessels.

Following delivery, hemorrhoids are due to obstetrical trauma and the great pressure that pushing the baby out exerts on the fragile blood vessels in the anal region. The initial tumescence (the blood clot caused by the ruptured vessel forms a bluish core) is accompanied by painful swelling. If a hemorrhoid is external (you can feel that the vein has erupted from the anus), you often can manually reinsert it. Sometimes, an anal fissure (a lesion of the anal canal, whose symptoms are intense pain during a bowel movement and bloody stools) accompanies hemorrhoids. The pain will diminish in the hours that follow but will return with the next bowel movement. An anal fissure that has not disappeared within six weeks after delivery needs to be treated by your gynecologist.

## How Long Do They Last?

Painful postpartum hemorrhoids can disappear within twenty-four hours . . . or remain for up to ten days. But piercing pain is not normal. Do not hesitate to consult your doctor if you experience such pain. The most important step in soothing hemorrhoid pain is to reduce the swelling.

**Anti-inflammatories**: These are usually topical, in the form of creams applied around the anus or just inside, with the help of a special applicator. Unfortunately, most creams sold over-the-counter are not very effective. Only prescription creams (which contain higher concentrations of cortisone) really seem to work. Don't hesitate to consult with your doctor about your hemorrhoids. Oral anti-inflammatories also can be prescribed, depending on whether you are breast-feeding. (In small doses, they may be prescribed during the twenty-four to forty-eight hours preceding your milk coming in).

**Sitz baths** can be helpful if you take them three times a day for four or five minutes, using cool water with a diluted antiseptic such as Witch Hazel.

According to Chinese medicine, hemorrhoids are due to a stagnation of cold energy (Yin) and heat (Yang energy) therefore is required to heal them. Acupuncture, especially when accompanied by *moxa* (a tiny bundle of slow-burning herbs that is lit and held a host distance from the skin), has a remarkable effect on hemorrhoidal swelling.

**Watching what you eat**: Preventing constipation is the name of the game and will permit you to avoid 75 percent of potential complications. Do not eat fatty products, and keep your intake of dairy products and animal protein down—try to eat red meat only once a week. New mothers who need to increase their calcium and protein intake can find a number of sources other than milk and red meat (see pages 137 to 138). Eat plenty of raw vegetables and especially fiber. Keep your fluid intake high: drink between 1.5 and 2 quarts of water per day. Finally, it is important to keep taking natural laxatives or stool softeners in a systematic way until your stools have been normal for two consecutive weeks. (Beware: Taking paraffin-based laxatives for

## HEMORRHOIDS

### Homeopathy

- 3 granules Aesculus 4C (Indian Chestnut) in the morning, 3 granules Collin Sonia 4C at noon, 3 granules Aesculus 4C before dinner, and 3 granules Collin Sonia 4C at bedtime.

    Aesculus is particularly recommended for strong, burning hemorrhoids. If your pain is dull but persistent, replace the Aesculus with Hamamelis (witch hazel) 5C.
- For hemorrhoids that ooze: 5 granules Graphites 5C three times a day or Sulphur 5C three times a day.
- To soothe itching and burning: 5 granules Fluoric Acidum 5C three times a day, or Carbo Vegetalis 5C if you are left with distended veins and a burning feeling after a bowel movement.
- If you have internal hemorrhoids only with backache, constipation, or bleeding: Calc Fluor 5C three times a day.
- If you have an anal fissure that is aggravated during bowel movements: 5 granules Nitricum Acidum, 5 granules, three times a day.
- For anal and perineal eruptions: 5 granules Hura Braziliensis three times a day.

### Herbal Remedies

- Yellow Dock, Dandelion, Nettle, and Oat Straw are all helpful in controlling hemorrhoids.
- Make sure that your diet includes plenty of garlic, onion, parsley, ginger, and dandelion roots.
- An infusion of Witch Hazel, Plantain, Marshmallow Root, and Oak Bark can be used on compresses to soothe burning and itching hemorrhoids. Pilewort ointment also is available in many health-food stores.
- Supplement your diet daily with 1 to 2 grams vitamin C.

several weeks can impoverish the body's supply of vitamins A, D, E, and K).

**Lifestyle habits also play a very important role**: Keep fit and avoid hot baths. Specialized pelvic floor exercises can soothe hemorrhoids by restoring proper circulation to the pelvic area.

## A COMFORTING POSITION

Lie down on your stomach (with a pillow under your head and another beneath your waist, leaving room for your breast in between) for 15 to 30 minutes a day. Rhythmically squeeze in your buttocks and release. This exercise will not do much to flatten your stomach, but it will soothe hemorrhoid pain.

If the hemorrhoids still do not disappear after you have tried all the methods recommended above, you should not hesitate to discuss with your doctor the advisability of having them surgically removed (either through cryosurgery—freezing or injecting them with liquid nitrogen—laser surgery, or by injecting a chemical to shrink the enlarged vein).

Hemorrhoid pain can be tiring and depressing. Do not hesitate to consult a proctologist, who can prescribe medications that are more effective than the over-the-counter variety. If necessary, this specialist can perform a minor surgical procedure or cauterize the blood vessels.

Preventing hemorrhoids from reappearing over time is a question of lifestyle and careful eating habits.

## After an Epidural

From 1981 to 1997, there was a tripling of the percentage of women in labor at large hospitals who had regional anesthesia, from 22 percent to 66 percent—notably epidurals. An epidural is the injection through a catheter of a novocaine-like anesthetic into the space around the *dura* (the membrane around the spinal cord)—not into the spinal fluid as is the case with the one-time spinal saddle block that our mothers may have had. It numbs the body from waist to toe, and allows for an almost pain-free labor and delivery (although in some cases, the anesthesia numbs only one side of the body or not at all). As labor progresses, the epidural may "wear off" and a woman will begin to feel some pressure during her contractions. When this occurs, the anesthesiologist may administer additional medication through the catheter. During the second stage of labor most women will experience some pressure while pushing, even with an effective epidural. This is necessary to allow women to assist with pushing. Increasing numbers of hospitals now offer "walking" or "light" epidurals, which provide pain relief while allowing you to move and fully participate in the second stage of labor. Epidurals are now often used for cesarean deliveries so that the mother can be awake to welcome her baby and avoid the unpleasant aftereffects of general anesthesia.

Despite its widespread use, the epidural (like the episiotomy) continues to be a subject of debate. Its supporters maintain that a woman who is more relaxed and less stressed during delivery will recover from childbirth more quickly. However, epidurals may contribute to the need for medical intervention during labor and delivery, in particular the need to stimulate labor with Pitocin. As with all forms of anesthesia, the side effects and potential complications of an epidural must be taken into consideration. Be sure to get the whole story before making a decision. An unmedicated delivery is both rewarding and possible with proper childbirth education and good support during labor.

## The Physical Aftereffects of an Epidural

The effects of the epidural anesthesia generally wear off within six hours. Sensation returns gradually to the legs, beginning with the toes. The most common physical side effects of an epidural are:

+ The expulsion phase of labor may last longer and can be less effective because the abdominal muscles have been numbed and cannot contract as strongly. Sometimes, the obstetrician must resort to using a vacuum extractor or forceps because of ineffective pushing. But with good prenatal training (childbirth education classes and appropriate exercises), a woman can participate actively in her delivery and diminish the risk of a forceps birth.

   More and more, the obstetrician or midwife will take advantage of "passive descent" during an epidural, when the contractions alone push the baby down into the birth canal without the assistance of the mother. Pushing is delayed in these cases until later in the second stage of labor.

+ Sometimes, when under epidural anesthesia, a woman may push and strain too strongly, subjecting her muscles to enormous stress. Again, proper preparation is important.

> To overcome the effect of anesthesia on the bladder, take one dose of Thebalcum 9 CH, to be repeated if necessary

♦ While an epidural is in effect, a woman may be lying for many hours in the same position, without realizing how uncomfortable or unnatural her position may be. She may unknowingly be stretching her ligaments, which are already weakened and distended as a result of pregnancy.

♦ During the expulsion phase, the baby puts pressure on the rear of his mother's pelvis (the sacrum), pushing it inwards. If she is lying on her back, especially if her legs are raised in stirrups, her coccyx (tailbone) cannot tilt back, as it should to let the baby through (while if the mother is vertical, the pelvis can expand up to 15 percent during delivery). The pressure caused by the baby's head moving through the birth canal can have repercussions on the entire spine, and may even displace the coccyx (see page 56). Over a third of women who deliver using an epidural experience difficulty with urine retention immediately after childbirth. The urethra, which is both anesthetized and compressed by the baby's passage, takes several hours or as much as a day to recover its normal functioning, even if it has not been damaged. It may therefore be necessary to drain the bladder with a catheter.

**Be sure that you at least try to void every two hours during labor and immediately after delivery. Keeping the bladder from "over filling" can prevent problems.**

When epidurals were first introduced fifteen years ago, serious side effects were more prevalent, such as debilitating headaches and dizziness when the catheter pierced the dura (spinal cord membrane), numbness in the legs if a small amount of the anesthesia reached the spinal fluid liquid, or sudden drops in blood pressure. Today, anesthesiologists have become so proficient and the epidural technique has been so perfected that these side effects have become quite rare.

## The Psychological Effects of the Epidural

Midwives note that new mothers who have delivered under epidural anesthesia sometimes feel a void, an impression of not having fully experienced one of the most important moments of their lives. This is doubtless due to the fact that since Adam and Eve, pain has been associated with childbirth—a badge of honor. A woman's aptitude to endure pain is almost synonymous with her ability to give birth. In our traditional imagery, the "good mother" is one who suffered in order to have her children. Even today when pain control has become a priority of the medical community, women continue to have mixed emotions about epidurals: they may fear the pain of childbirth, yet feel that using an epidural anesthesia amounts to resigning, to give up without trying.

On the other hand, because mothers-to-be are now told, "You have the right to not feel pain," they often think that they do not need to prepare for childbirth. As a result, many women who expected to sail effortlessly through an epidural-assisted delivery will discover that the human dimension quickly gains the upper hand. They may regret not feeling the baby's "passage." The anticipated progression from pregnancy to motherhood was interrupted, broken, and now, feeling a bit lost, they regret that they did not fully experience the moment of childbirth. Some women may subconsciously transpose that missed pain onto the postnatal period. According to midwives, it is probably for this reason that women today may experience far less pain in childbirth but complain much more of pain in the days that follow.

The epidural has also transformed another ancient rite: the role played by other females (mothers or midwives) in the childbirth process. Labor rooms are quieter. Midwives, who need to "accompany" mothers less and less often, are less involved in labor and can handle several patients at once. Midwives themselves say that when women do not complain, "we probably pay less attention to them." Another important change has occurred in the past thirty years: now that we are less vocal in our suffering, our partners have been allowed at our side during delivery. Childbirth has become an affair of the couple. But some women still feel (unconsciously, most of the time) the absence of a female presence as a large gap in their childbirth experience. Women should ask for the labor support they want. There is no reason why both their partner and a significant woman in their lives (mother, sister, or friend) cannot accompany them through labor and delivery.

## How to Overcome These Difficulties?

Do not forget that pain is not the determining factor in childbirth. Having an epidural does not mean you have not given birth. Live this moment to its fullest, with or without pain.

Even a delivery with epidural requires preparation. The epidural eliminates MOST pain, but does not change the way in which the baby is expulsed. Because you will have no sensation in the lower body, you will have to learn how to push properly so as not to damage your muscles and ligaments. This subject is covered in virtually all childbirth preparation classes.

If you have given birth previously with the aid of an epidural, and feel that you have overcome the fear of pain, you might try a second delivery without it.

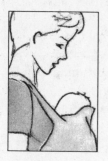

# 5

# After a
# Cesarean Section

Today, more than 20 percent of women in the United States deliver by cesarean section and many of these C-section births are scheduled. This proportion is higher than in most other industrialized nations, such as France, where the figure is close to 16 percent. The incidence of cesarean sections is on the increase for several reasons, including the rising age of many mothers, greater attention now paid to preventing fetal suffering, the fear of lawsuits, the growing number of twin and multiple births, and the increased number of induced births.

## The Operation

It is useful to know how a cesarean section is performed to understand its aftereffects. Most of the time, the incision is transversal, or horizontal ("Pfannensteil's incision"), and located just above the pubic bone, so that the scar will be hidden by pubic hair. Vertical incisions, from navel to pubic bone, have become exceptional and are used only in the most pressing emergencies.

The doctor makes a small incision through the abdominal wall, inserts retractors to hold the tissues open, and then separates the muscles. It is important to remember that the muscles are not cut. However, the doctor does cut through two layers of abdominal lining before reaching the uterus. The uterine wall is incised in the lower region (behind the bladder), which, having been stretched by the pregnancy, is now thinner. The amniotic sac is broken, and the baby's head appears. Amniotic fluid is sucked away with a tube. With the left hand the obstetrician extracts the baby's head while protecting its skull, and with the right hand pushes on the base of the uterus to help the baby come out. Then the umbilical cord is cut. Most of the time, the baby cries and is shown to his mother. Since most cesareans today are performed under epidural anesthesia, the mother is awake. Once the baby has been removed, the doctor detaches the placenta (or waits for it to be expelled naturally) and verifies that the uterus is empty. Finally, all the interior layers are stitched with self-dissolving thread. However, the skin may be stitched with nonabsorbent stitches, or even stapled together.

In the past, women were advised not to undergo more than three cesarean sections in their lifetime as the uterus used to be opened right in its center and the fragile scar tissues could not resist more than three operations. But with the advances made in surgical techniques and the practice of incising horizontally lower down where the uterine wall is more resistant, this limit is no longer necessary. The scar on the uterus is protected by the intestinal wall, bleeding inside the abdomen has been reduced to a minimum, and intestinal occlusions are now much less common.

It usually takes only eight to ten minutes between the moment the doctor makes an incision in the abdominal wall and the birth of the new baby. But the stitching of the uterine and abdominal walls takes some forty-five to sixty minutes.

After the baby is born and the placenta extracted, several medications are administered to the mother intravenously: synthetic oxytocin (also known as Pitocin) helps the uterus to contract; a morphine-based analgesic acts as a painkiller; antinausea drugs counteract any reactions to the morphine.

*A word of warning*: Morphine can affect the nervous system and actually worsen postoperative recovery. Some women find that morphine makes them extremely nauseous or causes skin rashes. If you have had previous unpleasant reactions to morphine, be sure to ask your doctor to replace any morphine-based painkillers with alternative drugs.

## General Anesthesia

If an emergency cesarean is performed after attempting a vaginal delivery without an epidural, the anesthesiologist may not have time to administer an epidural or it may be contraindicated. In this case, a general anesthesia is quickly administered. This happens in approximately less than 10 percent of cesareans.

Awakening from a general anesthesic can be painful. Trembling and shivering, confusion and agitation, vomiting and nausea are common reactions. It takes several hours to regain full consciousness, and therefore the first mother-infant contact will be delayed. It is very comforting during these difficult moments to have the baby's father by your side.

Because intubation (a tube inserted in the trachea during the operation to facilitate breathing) is often necessary under general anesthesia, many women wake up to a very sore throat.

### What Are All the Tubes for?

**The epidural catheter**: Some doctors will maintain a light epidural anesthesia for twenty-four to forty-eight hours to allow the new mother to walk and digest food without pain. However, the catheter can make the back feel sore up and down the spine. This is why many midwives report that women often ask for the catheter to be removed after twenty-four hours.

**An IV (intravenous tube)** makes it possible not only to nourish the new mother with water, sugar, salt, and other electrolytes (potassium, calcium, etc), but also to administer painkillers and antibiotics. The IV tube usually remains for up to forty-eight hours in order to give the digestive system time to resume its normal functions.

**A catheter** may be inserted up the urethra to empty the bladder and avoid fluid retention. It can remain inserted for several hours, or for up to two days if the bladder seems to have been traumatized during the operation, or if the woman is receiving anesthesia through an epidural. Since a urinary infection may occur when the urethra is catheterized (and occurs in 6 percent of cases), the medical staff will check regularly to ensure that urine is flowing into the Foley bag properly, and also check the urine's color. The catheter is only removed when the doctor is satisfied that enough urine of the right color is flowing and that there is neither retention nor infection. Once the bag has been removed, it may be difficult to urinate at first because of a lingering irritation caused by the catheter.

# Discomfort After a Cesarean

## Pain

Cesarean sections may cause a wide range of physical pain and discomfort. The day after a cesarean section is rarely the most painful, because most women are still on an IV and receiving pain relief. Furthermore, the intestinal tract is still dormant. The real pain will begin some forty-eight hours later, and then diminish between the third and seventh day after the operation. For these reasons, doctors use pain relievers (such as morphine) more and more frequently during the postoperative period. These medications will not be incompatible with breast-feeding because they are administered before the milk comes in. The baby absorbs colostrum in quantities far inferior to the milk he will receive later. Expect some discomfort associated with your cesarean to last about a month.

The good news however is that women who have their babies by cesarean section have fewer problems with post-pregnancy acne, fewer hemorrhoids, less vaginal discomfort, less discomfort with intercourse, and less difficulty reaching orgasm.

**Sore shoulders** are due to a pocket of air left in the abdomen during the operation. The air presses on the diaphragm and on the phrenic nerve, which reaches to the shoulders.

**Nausea** can result from the morphine contained in analgesics (painkillers). As vomiting is very painful after surgery on the abdomen, the doctor also may administer an antinausea medication intravenously.

**After-pains** (uterine contractions while the uterus is returning to its pre-pregnancy size) hurt because they affect a scarred uterus that is more sensitive. They are particularly painful during the first two days of breast-feeding, because the baby's suction on the nipples stimulates uterine contractions. Painkillers administered intravenously can reduce

## A FEW WORDS OF ADVICE

When the uterus undergoes a contraction, try not to tense your body because tension increases pain. As soon as a spasm occurs, exhale deeply while trying to relax your abdominal muscles as much as possible. This requires full concentration. If you are in the middle of a conversation, do not try to be heroic: stop speaking, close your eyes, and think only of your body.

When lying down: Let your body go limp, and breathe deeply while concentrating on releasing your abdominal muscles.

When standing: Lean forward and go limp. Support yourself against a wall or, better yet, on a pillow placed on the tray table above your hospital bed. Close your eyes. Breathe slowly in a rhythmic manner, concentrating on your breathing and on relaxing your abdominal muscles.

When trying to get out of bed: If a nurse is present, lean on her and let yourself go completely. If you are alone, put a pillow on the tray table over your bed and lean on it.

this pain (if the new mother is breast-feeding, she may only be given painkillers until her milk comes in).

**Itching and skin eruptions** can affect women who have a cutaneous reaction to morphine. If you suffer from this, ask the nurses for a soothing lotion or apply compresses of witch hazel.

**Phlegm** may accumulate in your chest after a general anesthesia. Because coughing is painful while the abdomen is healing, women tend to suppress this natural reflex. To help relieve the need to cough, the following exercise is helpful: place a soft pillow against your stomach; inhale deeply; bend your knees up to your chest; exhale hard, like a steam engine; spit.

## When the Intestinal Tract Goes Back to Work

Anesthesia slows down the intestines, which provokes an accumulation of gas. Some women consider gas pains to be the most painful aftereffect of a cesarean section. This is why your first meals will be light (usually tea and crackers the first day, broth the next, and then the first meal on the third day). Your diet will progress based on how you feel and how your bowel reacts to the surgery. Your doctor will listen to your abdomen with a stethoscope for bowel sounds.

## *What You Can Do*

To eliminate gas:

- ✦ Drink a glass of very hot herbal tea with the juice of half a lemon.
- ✦ Practice one of the exercises recommended for constipation or backache (see pages 46 to 47 and 57) or one of the exercises below.
- ✦ Inhale and exhale by blowing like a locomotive (the same movement as for eliminating phlegm or mucus).
- ✦ Massage the abdomen, moving downward from the ribs to the groin, starting on the right side, continuing on the left, while imagining that you are pushing the gas through the large intestine and out.

### *Exercises for Eliminating Gas*

To be done while lying down five times in a row, several times a day:

- ✦ With your knees bent and feet flat on the mattress, hip-width apart, inhale slowly while extending the left leg. Let your foot slide along the sheet until the leg is flat on the bed.
- ✦ Exhale and bring the leg back to the bent position. Do not contract your abdominal muscles, just let the foot slide on the sheets while exhaling.
- ✦ Repeat both steps with the right leg.

(If you are afraid of being embarrassed by gas problems, ask your friends to wait two or three days before coming to visit you in the hospital.)

## Making Yourself Comfortable

**Lying in bed**: Try not to remain for too long in a half-seated position with your knees bent. If you are in this position, put a pillow under your knees. This is the most comfortable position, because it pulls the least on your stitches, but it promotes muscular laziness. Some practitioners advise the following position when you are lying down: keep one leg extended and one knee bent and up, with the foot flat on the mattress. Be sure to switch legs from time to time.

**To get out of bed or of an armchair**: Lean forward, keeping your back straight, until your feet support your body's weight. Then stretch your legs and bring your buttocks forward.

**To sit down**: Do the reverse—bend your knees, keeping your back straight, lean forward, place your hands on the seat, and back into it until you can put your bottom on the chair. Some practitioners recommend tying the sash of a bathrobe to the foot of your bed and hoisting yourself hand-over-hand when you want to sit up. This is much easier than using the trapeze that hangs over most hospital beds, which is generally placed too high to be useful.

**To lie down**: Face the bed, then get on it by crawling on all fours.

**To stand up**: It is very tempting to lean forward while holding tightly to your stomach and legs, but this position is tiring for the abdomen. It is better to stay as straight as possible. Even if this is harder in the beginning, the pain will go away more quickly if you make this effort.

## Getting Out of Bed for the First Time

You must get out of bed about twelve hours after the cesarean in order to avoid circulatory problems. This is probably the most unpleasant moment of the postnatal period. But it is absolutely necessary. One or two nurses will guide and support you. They will arrange your intravenous tubes, drain, and catheter so that you can take a few steps without disconnecting them.

Start by just sitting up. Pull one knee and then the other toward your chest while exhaling, sliding your feet along the mattress as though your knee were attached to a string. It is important to avoid putting pressure on the kidneys and stomach. Then roll over on to your side, rolling your body from head to toe as though it were all one block, and leading with your head and shoulder. Once you are on your side, gather your knees up as much as possible, and push yourself up with your arms.

Once you are seated on the edge of your bed, if the bed is not electric and cannot be lowered, be sure to ask for a footstool on which to place your feet. Slide your buttocks to the very edge of the bed. Then slide around, supporting yourself on your hands, until your legs are hanging over the side of the bed. Put your feet on the stool, straighten up, and, above all, do not look at the ground.

Take a few steps. If you are not receiving intravenous painkillers, you will probably be doubled over in pain by now, from the cesarean scar and from uterine contractions. Cross one arm over your stomach to hold on to the scar while you walk.

Try to stay as straight as possible. The more you move and walk, the faster the wound will heal, and the fewer complications there will be.

If a spasm starts, lean on the nurse and close your eyes. Concentrate on your breathing and on relaxing your abdominal muscles.

And then? Each day you will walk more easily, but you should not maintain a standing position very long. You can practice the very gentle exercises recommended on pages 79 and 81, which help to restore balance in the pelvic area and center your body.

## The Scar

The scar will become very sensitive, and will pull and itch. By contrast, the skin around the scar will seem numb. The stitches on different layers of the abdomen will not all heal at the same speed, so the differing tensions may cause some layers to pull a bit on the others.

Many women feel burning and itching sensations. When the pubic hair grows back in, it also irritates this area. Occasional pain and burning sensations can last for six to eight weeks.

### Caring for the Scar

The doctor or nurses will remove the bandage the day after surgery. This will allow them to monitor the healing process for any sign of infection. A cesarean scar has an advantage over an episiotomy scar in that it is in a drier and relatively sterile area. But it can become infected. If it is infected, it will become red and swollen, and it may pulsate or ooze some pus. It will also cause a fever. The doctor will immediately prescribe antibiotics. So as to avoid infection, try to follow the following rules of hygiene:

- ✦ Always wash your hands (preferably with disinfectant soap) before touching the wound or the bandage.
- ✦ Dry your hands with paper towels, because cloth towels harbor germs.
- ✦ Follow the instructions of the doctor who removes your stitches or staples. This is usually done before you leave the hospital.

## RECOVERING FROM
## A CESAREAN SECTION

### Homeopathy

The following pre- and postoperative homeopathic treatment has been proven to help patients recover their digestive functions much more rapidly than a classic allopathic treatment (see page 71).

- For two or three days before surgery: 2 granules Arnica 5C morning and evening.
- The day before the cesarean: 1 dose Arnica 9C on an empty stomach.
- The morning of the surgery: 1 dose Gelsemium 9C, 1 dose Arnica Montana 9C, and 1 dose China Rubra 7C.
- After the operation: 1 dose Arnica Montana 15C when you return to the recovery room, if possible (you may have to wait until you are in your room again). Then Opium 25C in the afternoon and Staphysagria 12C in the evening.
- The next day: 1 dose Arnica Montana 15C and Opium 30C in the morning.
- For one week after the cesarean: 2 granules morning and evening of each of the following Arnica Montana 5C, Gelsemium 5C, Pulsatilla 5C, China Rubra 5C, and Staphysagria 7C.
- To prevent postoperative swelling, 3 granules Apis 9C twice a day.
- To ease digestion, or in the case of pain and bloating due to constipation, take Raphanus 5C every two hours until you are able to pass gas, then three times a day until you have normal bowel movements again.

### Herbal Remedies

- Valerian tea, taken three times a day, helps overcome the pain of a cesarean incision.

## Exercises

It is essential to practice breathing exercises after a cesarean. Even if it hurts in the beginning, exercise will prompt the abdominal muscles to recover their tone more rapidly and will speed up the healing process as well. Here are a few useful exercises in addition to those recommended for women who deliver vaginally.

+ Hold a soft pillow against your stomach, breathe deeply while concentrating on your breathing and bending your knees. Blow hard, like a locomotive. This exercise is particularly recommended for controlling gas pains and eliminating mucus in the lungs.
+ Sit on your bed with your feet stretched out. Stretch your toes out, trying to bend them toward you, and then bend them away from you. Repeat this twenty times energetically so as to stimulate circulation. You can do this with both feet together, or one after the other. Vary the pattern so you don't get bored.
+ Separate your legs and rotate your ankles one direction, then the other.
+ Press the backs of your knees into the mattress, then relax. This makes your thigh muscles work and improves circulation.
+ Lying on your back, bend your knees (by sliding your heels along the mattress so your knees rise gently), then curl your pelvis up as if you wanted to roll your tailbone into your stomach. Hold this position for four seconds, then relax. Repeat this as often as you can throughout the day.
+ After the stitches have been removed: Lie on your back, bend your knees, feet flat, hip-width apart. Let your knees fall together to one side, then to the other, by "rolling" on your buttocks.

## The Baby Born by Cesarean

If the baby is healthy, you may begin to nurse him in the recovery room.

A woman who has prepared herself during pregnancy for the possibility of a cesarean can remain emotionally very close to her baby. Most childbirth classes do broach this subject since more than 20 percent of babies are now born by this route. If they don't talk about cesarean births in your class, be sure to ask. If she is not prepared, when an operation is necessary, a woman may experience disappointment and regret, or even feelings of failure for not having delivered the baby conventionally. She may feel a sense of guilt that the delivery did not go as expected or that she did not exercise enough control over the birthing process. Yet it is important to remember that each one of our birth experiences is unique and may only remotely resemble a traditional model of birth and motherhood. Each woman must embrace her experience as her own.

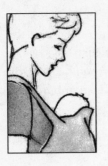

6

# Reclaiming
# Your Body

**M**any people still believe that a new mother should not exercise for forty days following childbirth. This misconception dates from the days when "getting back into shape" consisted only of abdominal gymnastics. Breast-feeding and the continued presence of pregnancy hormones are also given as excuses for delaying exercises that will help the body recover its pre-pregnancy equilibrium. We tend to forget how important it is for a new mother to "reclaim" her body after childbirth.

This renewal process serves a psychological purpose as well. The sooner a new mother acknowledges the changes brought on by pregnancy, the sooner she will be able to begin the restoration process. Armed with the confidence found in taking control, many women will feel better equipped to meet the challenges of motherhood while they also will avoid any further damage to their bodies.

After childbirth, the abdomen appears distended and flabby. Many women feel a sensation of "emptiness" inside. In order to "fill" the emotional and physical gap left by the baby, a mother needs first to regain consciousness of her lower body, then to tone and strengthen all of the weakened muscles. Two very gentle exercises should be started the day after a vaginal delivery or three days after a cesarean section.

## Rehabilitating the Pelvic Floor Muscles

If you are not aware of the vital importance of the pelvic floor to a woman's health and well-being, we recommend that you first read Chapter 23.

During pregnancy, hormones loosened the pelvic floor muscles, and childbirth then made them rigid as their fibers were stretched. It is therefore extremely important first to relax these muscles, thus restoring their balance before attempting to gently tone and strengthen them. An episiotomy scar or a tear should not prevent you from practicing these exercises, which in fact may well be less painful than many other normal functions. Gentle movements will allow you to realize that, despite your apprehensions, these muscles can move and contract without pain. Alternating movements of tension and relaxation will allow excess blood and other fluids to drain from the tissues. This in turn will contribute to a faster healing of bruises and hematomas. Your scars will become suppler through these exercises and will benefit from the increased blood supply to the area.

### Exercises

This exercise is the first step towards healing the pelvic floor muscles: at this stage, it will serve more to regain consciousness of this area rather than actually tone the muscles.

Lie on your back, knees bent, concentrating on the pelvic floor. Try one or all of these three possibilities:

+ Pretend you are trying to suppress passing gas. The anus will contract. Then relax.
+ Pretend you are trying to interrupt your urine stream or hold back urine. The urinary sphincter will contract. Then relax. This is a Kegel exercise that you may already have learned in your childbirth preparation classes.
+ Squeeze the lateral walls of the vagina. Relax.

Whether you manage to move one muscle or several, the pelvic floor muscles are working. Concentrate just as much on the sensation of relaxing the muscles as you do on contracting them. Try not to confuse the pelvic floor muscles with those of the buttocks, stomach, or thighs. Sometimes you may be tricked by the effort you can feel. It is easier to contract these larger muscles, but in doing so you compress the pelvic floor and do not allow it to contract. The confusion happens easily unless you remember to think of this at the very beginning of each exercise.

## Recovering Pelvic Balance

The pelvis is a bony ring located at the bottom of the abdomen. At the front, the bones meet at the *pubic symphesis*. At the rear, they join with the base of the spine (the *sacrum*). The alignment of the pelvis determines the positioning of your entire body.

In early pregnancy, the fetus lies within this circle of bones. As the months go by, the uterus moves upward into the abdominal cavity so that the fetus may grow outside the bony ring. Under the influence of pregnancy hormones, the body's ligaments (tissues that connect bones) relax, permitting the pelvic bones to "open" for the baby's passage. They will not return completely to their original position, which explains why some women cannot fit into their old trousers even if they have lost all the weight gained during pregnancy.

A misaligned pelvis or a displaced coccyx (tailbone) will not only cause back pain but also pull on the pelvic floor muscles, which in turn will further aggravate the discomfort of an episiotomy scar or other abrasions caused by childbirth. The angle of the pelvis also affects the suspension of our internal organs. If the body is thrown out of alignment, the force of gravity will pull the internal organs into new, unnatural positions. But if the pelvis is repositioned properly, the woman's center of gravity once again moves towards the rear of her body, and her weight is distributed appropriately. The abdominal muscles are spared excessive strain and therefore can be toned more easily.

## Toning the Abdominal Muscles

As we discuss on pages 288 and 289, the pelvic floor muscles are much abused during pregnancy and delivery. But the abdominal muscles also bear a lot of strain. Between the fifth and seventh months of pregnancy, the *rectus abdominus* (the superficial muscles that run vertically on either side of the abdomen) stretch over six inches. Normally, these muscles are joined along a narrow fibrous strip. During pregnancy, this strip thins and stretches along with the stomach muscles to make room for the baby. Immediately after childbirth, you can feel a sort of soft, pulpy ribbon in the middle of the abdomen running from your navel to your pubic bone. For the first four days, you may be able to fit two fingers in the space between the rectus abdominus muscles. In most cases, the gap closes spontaneously as the muscles regain their tone. But for some women who have delivered twins, a very large baby, or have given birth several times in rapid succession, the muscles may be so weak that the internal organs can be felt pressing against the skin. In such situations, surgery may be required to mend the muscles. (For a more detailed discussion of this problem, please refer to pages 307 to 308). For these reasons, it is important to begin toning and strengthening the rectus abdominus muscles soon after childbirth.

## Exercise

+ Lie on your back, legs stretched out flat. Focus your mind on your lower back.
+ Bend your knees, feet flat on the floor, hip-width apart.
+ Place your hands on your stomach and feel the movement of your breathing. With your hands, follow the inhale and exhale: as you inhale, your stomach rises and your hands rise and separate; when you exhale, your hands fall back down and come together.
+ Continue the same movement while breathing more deeply (do not force your breathing).
+ Now bring your stomach in as far as possible without straining. You are guiding the stomach in the direction it needs to take to recover. This exercise will allow you to feel, little by little, that your belly is less empty, that you are reclaiming it for yourself.
+ Continue, while exerting light pressure with your feet against the ground, as though you want to push through the floor. Gently contract your buttocks. The pubic bone will rise, the lower back will flatten, and your entire back will stretch and

# A FEW TIPS FOR A
# CALMER HOSPITAL DEPARTURE

The day before you are to check out, send home as much as possible, especially flowers, plants, gifts, and any large items.

You probably will still be wearing maternity clothes—or at least ample, roomy clothes—for another two weeks. For the next two to six months, be prepared to wear clothes that are two sizes larger than your pre-pregnancy clothes.

When leaving the hospital, you will probably be escorted to the door in a wheelchair. Some hospitals allow you to walk to the door unescorted. Once you are released by the nurse or aide, carry only the baby and your handbag, and a burp cloth in case the baby spits up. Ask the person accompanying you home to carry everything else.

A new mother walks more slowly than usual, especially after a cesarean. Take your time.

Checking out of the hospital always takes more time than you think it will. If you are still taking painkillers, keep them handy, so as to be at ease on the way home.

Ask the person accompanying you to bring the car close to the hospital door.

If you have never put a baby in a car seat, do not underestimate how complicated this can be at first. You should have at least read the instructions beforehand and preferably practiced at home. Some mothers prefer to settle the baby into the car seat while still in the hospital, and then install the seat in the car with the baby already in place. Do not forget that you should never place the car seat in front of an airbag. Pediatricians also advise against leaving the baby in a car seat for several hours. Once on the road, resist the temptation to take the baby in your arms to comfort or feed him. If you must take him out of the seat, ask the driver to pull over to the side of the road.

In winter, ask your family to turn the heat up in your home to 72°F. the night before you come home, so that the temperature will be comparable to that of your hospital room. Once you are at home, you can reduce the temperature one degree every day until you reach your household's normal temperature.

To save your partner needless trips to the pharmacy, buy all your sanitary napkins ahead of time for the four to six weeks during which you will be bleeding (special postpartum, extra-long and extra-absorbent for the early days or "overnight" pads, then normal ones for day and night, and finally smaller pads for light flows).

Before leaving the hospital, ask for the direct number of the maternity ward and the name of a nurse or two (and their shift hours) that you can call from home if you have an important question. Many hospitals provide a call service or "warm line" for new mothers with questions.

relax. At the same time, your belly will tighten a little, and your pelvic floor will spontaneously move upwards.

This exercise is so gentle that you can practice it even after a cesarean. Although the abdominal muscles were forced apart and stretched (but not cut) you still may feel as if you have been "cut in half." By restoring balance to your pelvis, you will restore sensation in your body and you will feel your muscles become "whole" again. These exercises, which are not violent and require no intense muscular effort, are extremely beneficial after a cesarean section. They will allow you to center yourself; to reenergize and rebalance the intraabdominal pressures in a part of the body that has been immobile for many months.

## When to Practice the Exercises?

With an empty bladder, repeat these movements in small series. The force and the speed with which you conduct them are less important than getting the movement right. Each practice, try to exercise for a little longer time and with a little more force, so that the muscle will not only move, but will actually become toned. In the beginning, you may not be able to do an exercise more than five or ten times. Your goal should be to do a series of thirty, three times a day, by the sixth week after childbirth.

The first step towards getting back into shape is to become aware of your body and its new challenges during the very first days, while you are still in the hospital. The second step is to continue these exercises at home for at least six weeks.

In addition to these exercises, try to urinate regularly (between six and eight times a day).

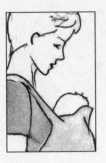

# 7

# Possible Postpartum Complications

Not only have serious postpartum complications become increasingly rare, when they do arise, they are now better handled by modern medicine. With proper monitoring during the prenatal months, doctors and midwives can identify high-risk women and can observe them closely in the days after delivery. New mothers also are better informed and know now how to interpret alarming symptoms. These complications fall into three major categories: infections, hemorrhages, and serious circulatory problems (thrombophlebitis and embolisms).

## Infections

### Infections of the Genital Organs

The primary symptoms are a foul-smelling discharge without uterine pain, accompanied by a fever of 100° to 101°F. Such infections are usually due to an infection inside a pocket of blood from a bruise caused by childbirth, torn perineal stitches, an infection of the episiotomy or tear scar, bad hygiene, or a preexisting vaginal infection.

This type of infection should be treated immediately with antibiotics so as to avoid further complications. Women generally are closely monitored after childbirth for this type of infection: the odor and appearance of blood on their sanitary napkins, as well as their temperature and blood pressure, are checked regularly. Once home, new mothers should continue to check themselves in the same way.

## Uterine Infections

"Child-bed fever," as described in nineteenth-century novels was, along with hemorrhages, the principal cause of death in childbirth for women right up until World War II. Today, however, this form of infection has become rare in Western countries, thanks to improvements in hygiene, better monitoring in hospitals, and the use of antibiotics.

Symptoms of uterine infection include foul-smelling lochia (postpartum bleeding), pain in the lower abdomen (including a very painful uterus) and lower back, fever above 101°F. for more than four hours, and a rapid pulse. While in the hospital, if any of these symptoms appears, the medical staff will take the woman's temperature and immediately administer antibiotics. In the most serious cases, symptoms of a uterine infection will appear within twenty-four hours following delivery. But it can also begin any time during the first three weeks.

In order to avoid infection, be sure to insert nothing in the vagina (especially tampons) as long as the cervix has not closed, that is, as long as you are still bleeding.

If a fever above 101°F. persists for more than twenty-four hours, call your doctor immediately.

## Urinary Infections

These are caused by germs in the urethra or bladder. Risks of urinary infection (*cystitis*) increase during the postpartum period for several reasons: the urinary sphincter remains distended for some time and cannot prevent some urine from dripping back into the bladder; a distended bladder may not be able to empty itself completely; a catheter may irritate the bladder; and the urethra may have become bruised during the baby's passage. Also, poor hygiene may lead to germs entering the urinary passages when a urinary catheter is inserted.

Urinary infections are identified by the following symptoms: a fever

## URINARY TRACT INFECTIONS
## (CYSTITIS)

### Herbal Remedies

The following herbs can be taken in an infusion: Marshmallow, Horsetail, Couchgrass, Cornsilk, Meadow Sweet, Nettle, Marigold, and Liquorice Root.

Another infusion to help boost the immune system is made with Purple Cone Flower, Marigold, Thyme, and Wild Indigo.

Drink plenty of unsweetened cranberry juice (available only in health food stores).

Compresses soaked in an infusion of Chamomile, Sandalwood, Bergamot, and Lavender may help relieve itching and burning due to a urinary tract infection.

Make sure to eat plenty of garlic—it is an excellent internal antiseptic.

### Aromatherapy

For benign urinary infection or cystitis: 2 drops essential oil of Sarriette and 1 drop essential oil of Lemon or Rosemary SB 1.8 on a sugar cube or in a spoonful of honey three times a day Mountain Savory (Satureja Montana sapmontana) is a powerful aseptic agent, highly recommended for intestinal and urinary infections.

### Homeopathy

If you feel an ineffectual urge to urinate or have problems with incomplete evacuation after surgery or a high tech birth: Staphysagria 5C three times a day.

over 101°F. (although it is possible to have cystitis without a fever), lower back pain (often on one side only), difficulty in urinating which lasts more than twenty-four hours, or an urgent need to urinate but passing only a small flow with a burning sensation (especially after any perineal scar has healed). Because the whole perineal area is sore in the days following delivery, a urinary infection can be difficult to detect. Classical medical treatment consists of a course of antibiotics after the type of bacteria present is identified through a urinalysis.

A urinary infection that is left untreated can lead to kidney infec-

---

**POSTPARTUM INFECTIONS**

The following alternative remedies are recommended in addition to hospitalization and conventional medical treatment.

*Homeopathy*
- Bryonia is recommended for any kind of peritoneal infection.
- Pyrogenium 200 is helpful for any infection of the genital organs or of the cesarean scar.

---

tion, which is far more serious, and which is characterized by a high fever and serious lower back pain that radiates down the legs, usually only on one side. This complication may need to be treated with intravenously administered antibiotics.

## Other Types of Infection

+ Local infections, such as an infection of the cesarean or episiotomy scars, are usually benign. Nevertheless, it is important to scrupulously follow the hygiene routine recommended in this chapter, especially if you are sharing a bathroom.

+ There may also occur infections, rare but serious, caused by obstetric trauma and characterized by an inflammation of the tissues of the lower pelvic region. They can spread to other organs of the body, such as the intestinal lining (*peritonitis*). Such infections can also occur after cesarean sections (and cause a high risk of intestinal blockage).

+ Rare, but serious infections may also occur that move to the bloodstream (*septicemia* or blood poisoning). These may start as a local infection, but the germs pass into the bloodstream. The symptoms are a very high fever with shivers, or hypothermia (a dramatic drop in body temperature). Immediate medical attention is crucial.

# Hemorrhages

Less than fifty years ago, women feared a postnatal hemorrhage as much as a uterine infection. With the advanced medical surveillance now given in developed countries, the risk to new mothers has been greatly minimized. But even today, hemorrhages remain the prime killer of women giving birth around the world.

Most often, a hemorrhage is caused by a placenta that has not fully separated from the womb and therefore not been fully expelled. It is the completed expulsion of the placenta that signals the body to compress its blood vessels through uterine contractions. This is why the midwife or doctor always examines the expelled placenta to make sure it is complete. Any piece of placenta or membrane left inside the uterus must be removed.

## Other Causes of Hemorrhages:

+ **Uterine atony** or inertia occurs when the uterus remains too "elastic" and does not respond to contractions. This can happen when twins, a very large baby, or excessive amounts of amniotic fluid have overly distended the uterus. It can also be due to a uterus that has become fatigued by repeated pregnancies. Sometimes; a very speedy delivery can cause "secondary inertia."
+ **A large tear in the cervix**.
+ **An overly full bladder** that gets in the way of uterine contractions.
+ **An infection** that hinders the contraction process.
+ **Serious clotting problems**.

With proper prenatal monitoring, these risks can be sidestepped and prevented with appropriate medicines.

## The Primary Hemorrhage

If a woman loses more than one quart of blood in the twenty-four hours following delivery, it is referred to as a primary hemorrhage, or delivery hemorrhage. This affects between 2 and 7 percent of women giving birth.

Between the baby's birth and the expulsion of the placenta, a trickle of blood runs from the vagina. Once the placenta is out, the empty uterus begins to contract and thus compresses a number of blood vessels. Often, a woman will receive oxytocin intravenously, so as to help the uterus contract. But if the bleeding continues or if the midwife or doctor notices that the expelled placenta is not whole, a uterine revision is necessary. In cases where the placenta has remained in the womb, they will perform a manual removal of the placenta.

If the woman is not already under an epidural, the doctor will administer a short-term general anesthesia, because manually stripping the placenta from the uterus is very painful.

## The Secondary Hemorrhage

In one case in two hundred, debris from the placenta that had been left in the womb will not be immediately visible. Suddenly, some twenty-four hours after delivery, or even two weeks later, the woman will begin to bleed profusely. This is called secondary hemorrhaging. The risk of infection is high in this situation (its symptoms are foul-smelling discharge, fever, and pain in the womb area).

How to recognize a secondary hemorrhage?

+ The bleeding will soak more than one sanitary pad every hour.
+ The lochia (postpartum bleeding) are still bright red, more than four days after delivery.
+ One blood clot the size of a golf ball or several clots larger than one inch in diameter are passed.

If you notice any of these symptoms, it will be necessary to perform a uterine revision, accompanied by injections of hormones that help the uterus to contract (oxytocin and/or prostaglandins), as well as treatment with blood thinners and antibiotics. A blood transfusion may be necessary. Fortunately, a woman's blood volume at the end of pregnancy is some 35 to 40 percent higher than normal. In Western countries, well-nourished women can afford to lose up to one quart of blood without serious consequences.

# Serious Circulatory Problems

Once the delivery is over, the body starts producing natural coagulants so as to prevent hemorrhaging. This coagulation capacity helps the uterus to stem the flow of blood at the site where the placenta was detached. But in the rest of the body, especially in the legs or in the pelvic area, blood can stagnate. If it turns into a blood clot, this can cause *thrombosis* (clots) or *phlebitis* (inflammation of the vein).

Midwives and nurses are trained to watch new mothers closely and to detect any sign of thrombosis. These include a fever of over 101°F., pain when the leg is stretched (such as pointing the toes), and heat and throbbing in the thighs and calves, with or without redness and swelling.

Getting out of bed soon after delivery is the best way to prevent phlebitis. For this reason, women who have had cesarean sections and must remain horizontal for 24 hours will be given blood thinners.

A new mother who suffers from weak veins should wear support hose, which are widely available in drugstores. (Choose the size for pregnant women, as your waistline will still be large).

Minor circulatory problems, notably migraine headaches due to the swelling of blood vessels in the head, also appear during and after pregnancy, triggered by high estrogen levels. About 18 percent of all women are prone to migraines. Of these, 11 percent had their first attack when pregnant for the first time.

---

## CIRCULATORY PROBLEMS

### Homeopathy

If you were already suffering from weak veins (varicose veins on the legs or vulva) during pregnancy, you can help tone your blood vessels by taking 3 granules Pulsatilla Nigerians 9C every two hours for the first 24 hours following delivery, and then three times a day during the days that follow.

### Aromatherapy

Take 1 drop essential oil of Cypress and 1 drop essential oil of Rosemary SB 1.8 on a sugar cube or in a spoonful of honey three times a day. Cypress acts as a decongestant and helps the blood vessels to contract.

## Additional Resources

The National Association of Mothers Centers (NAMC)
64 Division Avenue
Levittown, NY 11756
800-645-3828

Postpartum Education for Parents (PEP)
P.O. Box 6154
Santa Barbara, CA 93160
805-564-3888
*www.sbpep.org*

National Association of Postpartum Care Services (NAPCS)
2305 N.W. 37th Ave
Coconut Creek, FL 33066
800-453-6852
*www.napcs.org*

# II

# Your First
# Few Weeks

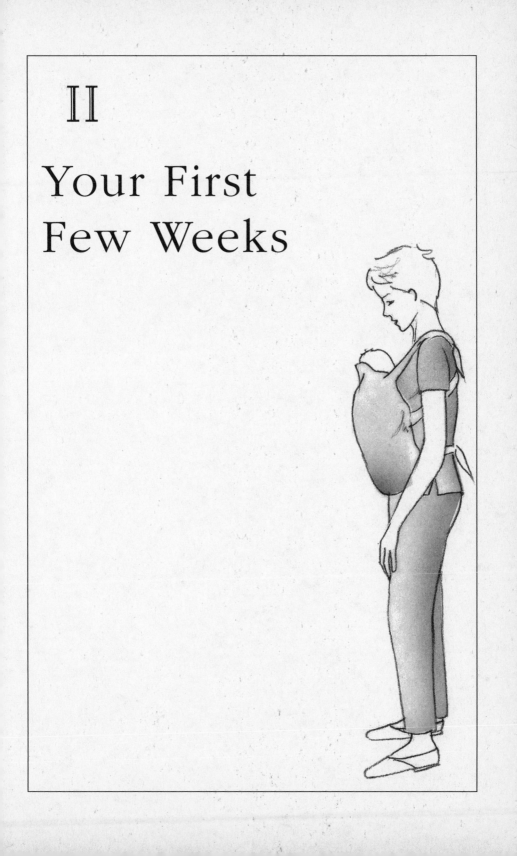

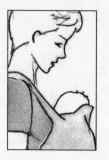

*8*

# A Changed Lifestyle

It happens time and again: a radiant mother is all smiles as she leaves the hospital with her newborn. Less than two hours later, she has collapsed into a heap of tears . . . Why? It's usually at this point that reality hits. She has left the reassuring cocoon of the hospital and now must face the demands of running a household, raising her other children, and caring for a new baby. She may be aching from her stitches, exhausted from lack of sleep in a noisy hospital ward, feverish from the arrival of her milk supply, or starting a bout of baby blues. But everyone around her expects life instantly to return to normal.

## Your Fragile Body

Arriving home with a new baby should not mean returning to an active life. Recovering from childbirth requires a period of transition, of "cocooning," because a mother's body needs at least ten weeks of rest and recuperation. It takes most women at least three months to feel fit again, but many need at least six or eight months. Why is this?

As we have seen in the previous chapter, the genital organs take six weeks to return to their normal size and function.

Postpartum bleeding (lochia) can last four to six weeks. Blood loss, combined with a slower blood circulation during the first two months, may lead to anemia, which causes fatigue (even if your hemoglobin levels were adequate during pregnancy).

Minor complications such as hemorrhoids, a displaced coccyx (tailbone), or episiotomy pain also cause discomfort and tiredness. Episiotomy and cesarean scars can ache for days, even weeks in some cases.

Your pelvic floor was distended, possibly even torn or cut during childbirth. Furthermore, the pregnancy hormones that loosen your muscles and ligaments will be present in your body for another three to five months after childbirth. As a result, the organs in your pelvic cavity, such as the lower intestine, colon, and bladder, will be less well supported by your pelvic floor. This explains why one out of three women suffers from "stress incontinence" (loss of a few drops of urine when coughing, sneezing, or laughing) in the days after childbirth. Other parts of your body, especially your abdominal muscles, also will have lost tone during pregnancy. All of the body's joints are more fragile. So for a few months after childbirth, you will be quite vulnerable to backaches. This is why it is particularly important to watch your posture during the postpartum period.

Extra weight, stretch marks, varicose veins, skin pigmentation, and some of the other demoralizing side effects of pregnancy can persist for several months after the baby's birth.

You may feel less coordinated for some time after childbirth and bump into things or accidentally cut yourself. Many new mothers are absent-minded—they'll dial a telephone number but forget whom they are calling; they'll start the washing machine without putting in the detergent; they'll lose their car keys. These lapses of attention are caused by sleep deprivation, hormonal changes, and simply "information overload."

Although breast-feeding is not in itself tiring, it does require total availability in the first weeks after the baby's birth.

You also are emotionally fragile. During the first eleven days after childbirth, eight out of ten women go through at least one bout of the "baby blues," a feeling of melancholy that can last from several hours to several days (see pages 210 to 215). At some point during the weeks

**HELPFUL HINTS**

In the past, women stayed in bed for twenty-one days following childbirth. Today, they are shopping for groceries three days after delivery. There is a happy medium between these two extremes. The following advice should help you recover faster and more effectively:

- Spend as much time as possible in the horizontal position. Before sitting down, ask yourself, "Could I do this lying down?" or if you need to stand, ask yourself, "Could I do this seated?"
- Don't carry anything heavier than your baby.
- Always pay attention to your posture—your back has never been so vulnerable.

following the baby's birth, nearly all new mothers will feel exhausted and overwhelmed. And for one in ten women, this emotional response will develop into a true "postnatal depression," a condition requiring psychotherapy and medical treatment.

So you've been warned! But you don't have to be one of the 64 percent of women who have bad memories of the weeks following childbirth. If you have organized these first few weeks before your delivery so that you can limit your daily chores almost entirely to the care of the baby, if you rest enough and nourish yourself well, you will give your body and mind the chance to regain their strength and equilibrium. Most importantly, you will be able to enjoy more fully the wonderful little being that has just entered your life.

## Getting Your Routine Under Control

Having a baby completely changes the way you use your time. That's how nature ensures that you'll have your priorities right—at least for a while.

As more and more women delay motherhood until they have proved themselves professionally, they grow accustomed to a well-ordered life: an established routine, coupled with moments of spontaneous leisure. Babies, however, cannot be managed in the same way.

They make huge demands on your time. In fact, for some time after his birth, it seems that the baby is "in charge." As obstetric physical therapist Christine Hill writes, "Babies have a well-developed capacity to elicit good parenting in order to survive." Through the power of his sheer helplessness, through his cute looks, through the enormous love that you will feel for him, your baby will ensure that you are at his beck and call. So how will you juggle his needs, as well as those of the rest of the family, of your household, and, in a few weeks, of your job?

In an ideal world, mother and baby should step into a bubble and live completely according to the baby's rhythms. For the rest of the family, it would be the equivalent of a mother leaving on a three-week trip, having organized everything in advance, so that the household could function without her. Although completely unrealistic in today's world (in any case, the baby's father and siblings have important roles to play), this image is useful to keep in mind.

## A New Lifestyle

Most mothers systematically place the needs of their children and of their mates before their own. In the long run, a mother who doesn't take care of herself will not take good care of her family. As a result, the irritation and frustration that she may feel at not being "the best" will take its toll on her patience and gentleness. She may even feel resentful towards the very children that she cares for above all else . . . You can avoid falling into this vicious circle by accepting the following realities.

## You Are Not a Superwoman

Becoming a mother requires a whole new perception of your time—it no longer belongs to you. The usual divisions of the day—morning, afternoon, evening—disappear. Work is never finished. The challenge is not to find a set formula but to learn how to juggle all the demands.

### Choose Your Battles
When a baby arrives, you'll have to choose your battles: set priorities and make sacrifices elsewhere. This is the secret to managing stress. According to Gillian Fletcher, a physical therapist who specializes in postnatal recovery, stress results from an "imbalance between the

## HELPFUL HINTS

Determine ahead of time how you and your partner will share responsibilities. You know your partner: his habits are not going to change overnight with the arrival of a baby. It's better to be pleasantly surprised when he pitches in more than expected, rather than angry and resentful when he doesn't live up to your expectations.

Be realistic about the time that each task will take.

From the start, establish times when you will be alone with your partner.

Always ask yourself: "Could someone else do this? Does it really have to be done?"

demands placed upon us in any situation and our ability to cope with those demands. The key factor here is our own 'perception.' " Rather than be a passive victim of circumstances, you can evaluate the importance of each situation and respond accordingly; this means that you are in control. As a new mother, you will be constantly confronted with difficult choices. For example, the baby is finally asleep. Should you take the opportunity to straighten up the house and throw in a load of laundry or should you take a nap?

## Manage Your Expectations

A woman who had a well-established professional life before the baby's birth, who thought that she knew how to manage and organize every facet of her routine, may find the constraints of life with a baby difficult to accept. During her pregnancy, she may have pushed her body by trying to overcome its physical limits. If she keeps this up after her delivery, she probably will take on too much. A vicious cycle of excessive expectations and disappointments sets in, which inevitably leads to frustration and resentment.

## Enjoy the Baby!

The first months with your new baby are precious and irreplaceable. Taking advantage of this new being should be your first priority, the ultimate goal of all your efforts.

Babies go through growth spurts during which their usual rhythms are upset, especially their feeding patterns. If you are breast-feeding, your breasts will need about two to three days to increase their milk production. These growth spurts usually occur at about:

> 6–10 days
> 3 weeks
> 6 weeks
> 3 months
> 6 months

Be prepared for these difficult days. This is not a good time to face other disruptions or to plan a trip.

## Organizing Your Return Home

It's easy to become discouraged by the sheer magnitude of the baby's needs. The best way for you to meet the needs of the baby and to find a little time for yourself is to learn how to manage your daily routine. Christine Hill writes that a new mother's ability to anticipate, to plan, and to organize before the delivery (rather than to react after the fact) is critical to having a satisfying postnatal experience. In any case, most women have no desire to make important decisions or to worry about anything beyond simple housekeeping at this time. They would love to be able to delegate all the logistic and managerial tasks of the household. All the more reason to plan in advance. You'll need:

### Help with Household Tasks
While you are in the hospital, and during your first week at home, you should avoid shopping, laundry, or housework. Neither should you walk the dog or take the children to school.

### Help During Your Rest Times
Whether it's for the entire night, every other night, or even in the afternoons, you will need regular periods of uninterrupted sleep. Once breast-feeding is established (see Chapter 15), someone else can change the baby's diaper and give him a bottle of expressed milk while you are sleeping.

**HELPFUL HINTS**

Make quick and easy meals—buy high-quality ingredients and prepare them as simply as possible. Pick foods that can be cooked together rapidly or that can be fixed in advance and cooked by someone else (casseroles, stews, sautés).

If someone offers to cook for you, don't hesitate to ask for the shopping and the dishwashing as well.

As soon as you feel up to it (and can organize a baby-sitter) go out with your partner for a quiet meal.

This is the time to do as much shopping as possible by telephone, from catalogues, or through the Internet.

### Help with the Older Siblings

If the children are old enough to play at a friend's house, ask the friend's parents to pick them up from school or to take them for a mealtime. Organize a network of baby-sitters who can take your older children out. It's a good time to spoil them with a special outing or a meal in a restaurant. But be sure to spend some time alone with them as well. Psychologists advise against sending siblings away to stay with friends or grandparents, unless the baby is born during a holiday period when the children would ordinarily be away from home. Try to fill their time with activities in addition to their normal routine. This means finding out ahead of time about schedules, transportation, and other logistics.

## The Right Kind of Help

Fortunately, most new mothers don't need medical care. What they do need is someone to help them with household tasks, to prepare meals, and to help care for the older children. Your partner can help with much of this, but his main task is to take care of you. So it's important to choose your help well. As this may take some time, it should be one of your priorities in the days and weeks before delivery.

## Your Mother or Mother-in-law

If you already have a difficult relationship with your in-laws, this is not the time to bring tensions into your home. Later on, however, your baby may provide a bridge between the two families.

It is often tempting to delegate household tasks to your mother or mother-in-law, and to concentrate on the baby. But your mother/mother-in-law may have her own habits and ideas about housekeeping. Are you ready to let her do it her way, at least for a while?

Be aware of potential conflicts between the two grandmothers. Sometimes the grandmother who has not come to help you is envious of the grandmother who has stayed with you.

Your partner may find it harder than you do to put up with his mother or mother-in-law under his roof. Try to determine ahead of time if her presence will be a source of conflicts in your relationship.

## Your Partner

The Family and Medical Leave Act of 1993 (FMLA) grants all workers (men and women) in companies of fifty or more employees up to twelve weeks of unpaid time off in the first year after a baby's birth to care for the baby. Although this act made millions of fathers eligible for paternity leave, less than 20 percent of those eligible have actually taken time off. Many fear that they can't afford to lose a paycheck, or that they may appear not to be committed to their career. If your partner does plan to take over household duties upon your return from the hospital, do remember that many women find it difficult to delegate to their partners. These mothers often seem to end up feeling more tired than those who had chosen other kinds of help. Their partners also complain about being exhausted. Unfortunately, when it comes to housekeeping, most women still feel that they need to explain and supervise everything (of course, you could be one of the lucky ones . . . ).

If your partner does not seem to have gotten the message that you need extra TLC, show him your lochia. Men seem to understand the connection between blood loss and weakness. . . .

## A Baby Nurse

If you are financially comfortable enough to afford one, a baby nurse can be a valuable source of information and expertise. They are a good solution for women who do not plan to breast-feed and who want to be able to sleep through the night. However, baby nurses rarely will help with household tasks (in the worst case, you may find yourself cooking for this helper). Baby nurses sometimes have difficult relationships with the older children. Therefore, it is essential to interview a potential baby nurse in your home before hiring her. Be sure to contact her references.

### A Doula

A wonderful source of support, doulas are becoming increasingly popular in the United States. Usually a woman, a doula assists the mother through labor and then offers in-home care during the early postpartum period. A doula eases the transition into motherhood by providing emotional support, along with breast-feeding advice and newborn-care tips. She also helps with household chores and the care of any older siblings.

### A Support Network

As a rule, your money will be better spent in hiring extra house help for shopping, cooking, and caring for your other children. Building a network of friends and family to whom you can assign tasks ahead of the baby's birth is the most important step you can take. Such a network will allow you to rely on more than one person. Female friends who already have children tend to be particularly supportive, because they understand a new mother's need to be pampered.

Before the baby's birth, draw up a list of names and equip yourself with a calendar. Contact friends in advance, asking them if they will help with specific tasks: household chores, baby-sitting, or even just dropping by for a cup of tea. This may mean a lot of phoning and advance planning, but the peace of mind it will bring you when you really need it is well worthwhile.

### The Pediatrician

One of the key figures in your network is your pediatrician. Choose him/her carefully before the baby's birth. Ask your family doctor, your obstetrician, and your friends. Take the time to interview him/her. Does he/she inspire confidence? Do you agree with his/her attitudes towards returning to work? Is there a lactation consultant on staff?

**HELPFUL HINTS**

If possible, test your "team" in advance. Choose people who know your house and your children well, whom you can trust, and who can provide you with emotional support.

Spread out your help. If your mother or mother-in-law offers to come for a few days, have her arrive after your partner has gone back to work. Avoid mixing too many generations under the same roof.

Delegate boring tasks; keep the fun ones for yourself.

Don't treat the person who comes to help you as a guest. They have come to help, not to be entertained.

Other people can't read your thoughts. Don't hesitate to tell those around you that you need help. Why not suggest that your good friends offer you baby-sitting time or grocery shopping instead of yet another baby gift?

Many pediatricians' offices now have office hours routinely on the weekend, as well as around-the-clock coverage. You may also find it useful for the office to have a regularly scheduled call-in time for casual questions about your baby's care and well-being.

## Relationships Change

A new mother's life is always centered on her baby. Your current circle of friends will be confronted by this new relationship. However, childless friends may not always realize how much upheaval you are experiencing. Conversely, your friends may see you only in your maternal role and may forget the person that you were before you gave birth. You may end up feeling as if your IQ has suddenly dropped. In reaction, some women feel obligated to prove to their friends, and especially to their colleagues at work, that they have not changed and can still compete at the same level. These attitudes obviously don't do much to foster the network of support and understanding that is so important for all new mothers.

Many new mothers suddenly find that they have less in common with friends who don't have children. Yet these same friends can be a valuable source of information and stimulation outside of family life;

they help keep your horizons open. Keeping close ties to women who don't have children or whose children are grown is especially important for the mother who stays at home and who may feel like she is losing her identity. The "stay-at-home-mom" often is excluded from social activities that strengthen and reaffirm her individuality and she is left feeling like she is only "the mother of . . ." or "the wife of . . ." This is why it is so important to take part in artistic, cultural, and social outlets that allow you to be creative, to develop your talents, and simply to have fun.

You'll need to explain to your friends that you value your time with them, even if these moments are less regular and spontaneous than before.

## Visitors

The arrival of a new baby always triggers an overwhelming response. All sorts of family, friends, and even the most remote acquaintances seem to appear out of the woodwork. A mob of visitors will crowd into your hospital room and into your home in the days following the baby's birth. Then you are deserted. Yet, even the proudest new mom may not feel like serving drinks to swarms of visitors. And most newborns are not thrilled at the prospect of being picked up and bounced, but simply

### HELPFUL HINTS

Take the phone off the hook or turn on an answering machine with a message about the newborn (name, weight, etc.) and suggest specific hours when you can receive calls (preferably when your partner is home).

About two or three weeks after coming home, organize a few afternoons of visits so that you can see one or two people at a time. Ask friends and relatives to let you know before they come. Warn them that they should plan to stay only for a short time.

Make certain that visitors don't smoke inside your home. Ask them to speak quietly.

If you feel uncomfortable breast-feeding in front of visitors, ask them to leave or to entertain themselves with television or magazines while you breast-feed in another room. Don't feel rushed. Your baby is your first priority.

want a chance to adjust to their new life outside the womb. So, with the obvious exception of your most immediate family and closest of friends, try to encourage all other visitors to wait a few weeks until you have regained your strength and your routine is under control.

## Siblings

Many mothers worry about the reaction of their older children when a new baby arrives. Everyone seems to have an opinion about how to prepare siblings for the birth of their little sister or brother. If you only listen to one piece of advice, remember this: it is the baby who needs to fit into your family's life, not the other way around!

Depending on his/her age and position in the family, each child will view the arrival of a younger sibling in a different way. A two- or three-year-old does not really understand what a baby is. Maybe someone has said that he would have a playmate and he is disappointed that the baby cannot play right away. Other children may interpret the baby's arrival as a punishment for their misbehavior: a new baby has stolen Mommy's time and attention.

Fortunately, a mother's capacity for love is limitless. Maternal love is not divided into little parcels, but simply increases with the arrival of each child. The ability of a mother to love her children is, however, quite a different matter from her ability to meet each of their needs. . . .

### Before the Delivery
If you are planning to put the older child in nursery school or day care outside your home, get him started well before the baby's arrival so that you may devote all the time he needs to become accustomed to his new routine. You may want to bring him to visit friends and relatives a few times so that you can organize outings for him in the first few weeks after the baby's birth. If your older children are home in the afternoons but no longer take naps, begin enforcing a "quiet time" after lunch so that you also may rest.

If your child's possessions or room will need to change to accommodate the baby, it's a good idea to do this at least a month in advance, whenever possible. If a sibling will have to move to a "big bed" in order to vacate the crib for the new baby, also try to make this transition as far ahead of time as possible. It's best to put away the baby bed for some time and to take it out again when the baby needs it so that the older child does not have the impression that the baby has stolen his bed.

Let your children participate as much as possible in the preparations for the baby's arrival. Some psychiatrists recommend having the older child choose a toy or piece of clothing for the baby that will be his "gift," as this gives the sibling the opportunity to be the generous "older brother."

### While You Are in the Hospital

Most children need to be reassured when their mother goes to the hospital: that Mommy has not disappeared, that she still loves them. It is even more important for your children to see you than to meet their new little brother or sister. Most hospital maternity floors have specific visiting hours when siblings are welcome. Try to arrange to have a friend or relative bring your older children for a visit as soon after delivery as possible. If that is not possible, your partner can take photos to bring home if you have access to a Polaroid camera or simply to a rapid-film-development center. Call your children daily to say that you are thinking of them and that you will be back soon.

Fathers, beware of letting your children sleep in bed with you if their mother stays in the hospital for several days—it will be difficult to wean them of this habit when she returns home.

### Coming Home

Some child psychologists advise parents to let the older siblings come to the hospital to escort the new baby to "their" home. If this is not possible, it is very important for the older children to be present at home when the baby arrives.

The baby's arrival is a difficult moment for the older child. He is no longer the family's sole center of attention. A very small child does not know how to say that he is jealous, but certainly feels that something has changed. Indeed, new mothers tend to be more impatient, more abrupt, and less readily available for their older children when there is a new baby in the family.

The first sign of discomfort may be troubled sleep (especially bothersome, as you will be waking anyway for feedings). Usually, if the child has negative reactions, they will be aimed at the mother in order to make her feel guilty. This tactic works quite well because most mothers will try to make amends towards their older children. (This is particularly true after the arrival of the second child—the effect fades a little after the third child.) He or she may wish for a time to become a baby again because everyone seems to be so concerned with the new arrival. This sort of regression (bedwetting, trouble sleeping, wanting to drink from a bottle) only means one thing: he wants care and attention. Other children may express their jealousy through aggressive gestures, sometimes directed at the baby. To protect the baby from physical aggression, do encourage verbal expressions of anger and never leave a toddler alone in a room with a baby. Explain to your older child that you would never have let anyone hurt him when he was a baby. Try not to be irritated by this jealousy; your child is already unhappy. What he really needs is your tenderness.

If the new baby is born from a second marriage, remember that a small child does not realize the difference between a half-brother and a full one. He must now share space with the newcomer. If the older child lives outside your home, be sure to reassure this child that he or she still has a place—his or her regular place—in the family.

The bond between siblings grows out of small gestures. A new baby also "belongs" to his or her older siblings who can share in his care: choosing his clothes, rocking the baby to sleep, singing songs, and helping with the bath routine. For example, when you sit down to nurse the baby, bring a few toys along for the older child so that he may play quietly by your side (some mothers find that this is a good time to read a story). Parents can say, "You see, he's really small, he doesn't know how to do anything, he has to be taught everything; will you help him since you already know so many things?" When the baby cries, you can ask your older child: "Do you think that he is hungry? Does she need to be changed? Do you think that it is hard for him not to be able to talk like us?" Focus on the positive and pleasant things that the child does for the baby: "Look at how much she likes you to stroke her back"; "look at how she turns her head when she hears your voice."

It is important to allow the older sibling to follow his usual schedule and to maintain a routine that it not invaded by the needs of the baby. Children need a routine; it reassures them. Above all, try to ensure that your preoccupations with the baby do not result in the older children being deprived of privileges granted before the baby's arrival.

The older sibling also needs moments that are his alone. Try to spend a few extra minutes with your older child whenever the opportunity arises. If he or she brings home a picture from school, don't just day "how pretty," but take the time to discuss it. Give advance warning to your children that you must attend to the baby rather than suddenly leave them in the middle of a game.

Finally, do what you can to prevent visitors from showing favoritism. Take them to greet the older children before showing them the newborn. And do try to avert the classic question, "So, are you happy to have a little sister (or brother)?"

## Pets

Pets can be as jealous as children can, especially if they played the role of the baby in the family. When the real baby arrives, many couples have less time for their pet, who may feel rivalry and compete for attention. What should you do?

Prepare the animal in advance as you would prepare an older child. If the pet is not house-trained, teach him before the baby's birth. Expose him to small children and babies as much as possible: encourage friends to visit with their children and babies in order to get the animal used to seeing children in his territory. Before the baby's arrival, don't refuse him access to the nursery. But once the baby is home do not let him in the room on his own.

During your hospital stay, your partner can bring home a cloth diaper that the baby has slept on, so that your pet can get used to the newborn's scent. Don't force it on the animal, just leave it around the house.

When you come home, continue to familiarize your pet with the baby's smell and encourage him to become friends with the baby. Pet him; speak to him in a gentle and encouraging voice. Neglecting an animal will only make him feel more rejected, so include the pet in family life as much as possible.

Don't put the baby's bassinet in a place where the pet could overturn it. Don't forget that even the cleanest pets carry dust and germs; don't let the animal jump on your lap when you are nursing or holding the baby. If you have a cat, either isolate him or always close the door to the baby's room, as cats love to curl up in cribs. After patting an animal, wash your hands before touching the baby, and change your shirt if it is covered with hair. (These precautions will become less important after several months when the baby's immune system is more mature.)

# Surviving Fatigue

You may feel that you are "back on your feet" just a few days home from the hospital. It is tempting to take on too much, but you risk collapsing a month later. Many new mothers experience a "crash" eight to ten weeks after the baby's birth, when the accumulation of sleep deprivation is at its worst. Remember that it is truly exceptional for a three-month-old to sleep through the night. Studies show that two-thirds of babies ages six to twelve months, and 30 percent of children one to three years old have trouble sleeping through the night. Michigan State University researchers have found that women who work and have children under the age of three get at least one hour less of sleep per night than their male counterparts. Just as a mountain climber begins ascending slowly at first to save strength for the final assault on the peak, a new mother must save her energy to avoid using up her reserves too soon. However, managing your time to make rest your top priority usually means a total reorganization of your normal routine.

We know that fatigue is inevitable during the postnatal period. Some sleep deprivation is almost unavoidable—but there is no need to suffer from utter exhaustion.

According to medical studies, the fatigue felt by a new mother reaches its peak two to four days after her return home—regardless of the length of her hospital stay. Only 50 percent of women feel that they have regained their usual energy levels by six weeks postpartum. Twenty-five percent more feel that they are back to normal after six months. This still means that a quarter of all new mothers suffer from fatigue and low energy more than six months after childbirth.

## Lack of Sleep

Most new mothers find that their biggest problem is lack of sleep. The sleep cycle is made up of four phases that in total last about ninety minutes. The last phase, deep sleep, occurs mostly early in the night. It is during this phase that physical recuperation takes place. Our immune system is more active when we sleep. Only after the full sleep cycle is completed can the body go into REM (rapid eye movement) sleep when we dream. REM sleep, which occurs principally later in the night, is essential for processing all the mental stimuli accumulated during the day. If a mother is woken during any stage within her sleep cycle, she will go back to the very beginning of the cycle again when she falls back to sleep and thus miss out on precious REM sleep. So even if a women is sleeping the same number of total hours within a 24-hour period as before her baby's birth, she may still suffer from REM sleep deprivation.

Elevated estrogen levels disturb the sleep patterns of many pregnant women. By the last weeks before their baby's birth, 68 percent of women also complain of trouble sleeping because of cramps, indigestion, hemorrhoids, difficulty breathing, or other discomforts of pregnancy. Seventy percent of pregnant women experience bad dreams or nightmares. As a result, many women are already quite tired when they arrive at the hospital to give birth.

Difficulty sleeping during pregnancy is due primarily to hormonal and physical causes and not to external factors such as the number of hours a pregnant woman works or the number of children she already has.

Because pregnancy hormone levels are still high in the first weeks after the baby's birth (especially when breast-feeding), sleep continues to be uneasy. Newborns sleep more lightly than older babies do: they wake easily and their rhythms are more erratic. Babies express their discontent at changes in their routine or surroundings through fussy behavior, including refusing to settle down.

If your baby has older siblings, their school schedule and activities also will make it more difficult for you to sleep. No sooner may you be settling back to sleep after an early morning feed, than it will be time to wake the older children for school.

Unfortunately, it's easy to accumulate a "sleep debt." Missing only seven or eight hours of sleep a week may cause the appearance of such symptoms as itching or burning eyes, blurred vision, chills, hunger for sweets and high-fat foods, and waves of fatigue. A lack of sleep will lead to irritability, lethargy, anxiety, and difficulty in concentrating . . . and a severe loss of sense of humor! As we will see on page 212, there is a close link between fatigue and depression. However, just two or three nights in a row of uninterrupted sleep can cure the symptoms of sleep deprivation.

Fatigue is managed by prevention: by building up energy reserves that can be called upon in times of stress, as well as never letting your-

## HELPFUL HINTS

- Try to take two naps a day, at least during the first few weeks after your baby's birth.
- Go to bed very early. When trying to try make up for lost sleep, it is better to go to bed early rather than plan to sleep late.
- As soon as the baby is sleeping, drop everything! Babies usually take their longest nap after a bath and feeding. Take advantage of this time slot!
- If this is your first baby, try to get everything done in the morning. But if you have older children, plan to sleep while they are in school.
- Organize your night feedings ahead of time. If you are breast-feeding and have the baby in bed with you or in a bassinet right by your bed, all you need to do is open your nightgown to feed the baby while lying down. Just anticipate what you might need to have on your bedside table (i.e., glass of water, clean diaper, and plastic bag for the dirty diaper). If you are not breast-feeding, and the baby has his own bedroom, feed him in that room. Prepare a comfortable chair with a blanket and extra pillows, a space heater (if the temperature in the room is under 70°F.), as well as all that you may need to change the baby. And don't forget to prepare a snack and a drink. Don't leave the main light on, as your baby needs darkness to learn to sleep as we do, but a nightlight will not be bright enough for you. So we recommend setting up a little lamp with a low-wattage bulb that will stay on all night.

self become completely exhausted. Airline pilots on long-haul flights will rest between legs of the journey. Surgeons rest between long operations. A new mother deserves the same treatment.

If you feel exhaustion taking over in the first few weeks or if your baby seems to be hungry every two or three hours, get help! Ask your partner or mother or hire someone (a student, for example) to come for part of the night or every other night to feed your baby expressed milk, so that you can sleep at least six hours in a row. Although it is not advisable to skip a night feeding when breast-feeding (so as to avoid engorgement and a drop in your milk supply), an exhausted mother's urgent priority is to overcome her sleep deprivation.

Sleep deprivation affects creative thinking, memory, and the ability to concentrate. Reaction time becomes slower and dangerous mistakes can be made. Therefore, avoid driving alone for long distances or

# FATIGUE

## Homeopathy

- On your return home: 3 granules Arsenica 9C three times a day.
- If your fatigue is accompanied by muscle cramps: 3 granules Cimifuga, Cuprum or Metallicum 9C every two hours until the cramps disappear, then three times a day.
- If your fatigue is "mental" and you have difficulty in concentrating: 3 granules Kalium Phosphoricum 9CH morning and evening.

## Herbal Remedies

- A relaxing herbal tea to drink at bedtime: mix equal parts of Linden, Verbena, Chamomile, and Passionflower. Use 1 tablespoon for each cup of water. Let steep for ten minutes.

## Aromatherapy

- For the treatment of insomnia: Two or 3 drops of essential oil of Lavender in your bath water or on your pillow.
- To fight fatigue: Mix equal parts of essential oils of Cinnamon, Lemon, Juniper, Mint, Rosemary, and Eucalyptus. Use 2 or 3 drops a day on a cube of sugar or in a spoonful of honey.

doing anything that requires concentration. The reflexes of a person who has slept very little over a period of twenty-four hours are as slow as those of a person who is legally drunk.

A newborn's sleep pattern depends above all on his weight. Low-weight babies are simply hungry more often. But you can start introducing a bedtime ritual early on. Just remember to stick to it. Children should grow up in a real world where people sleep at night, not just when they please.

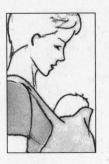

# 9

# Looking After Your Body

## Your Posture

### When Caring for the Baby

Adjust the crib mattress so that you don't need to stoop when picking up or putting down the baby. Most crib mattresses have adjustable heights and can be lowered as the baby grows and becomes more mobile. If the baby is in a bassinet, put it on a piece of furniture that is sufficiently tall and stable to save you from having to bend over.

Bend your knees when you pick up the baby from below your waist level.

Use a changing table that's the right height. If it's more than two or three inches below your waist (at the level of your hipbone), you will need to stoop when you change your baby. It's better for your back to change the baby on the floor (kneel on one knee) or on a bed (with you kneeling by the bed).

Adjust stroller handles so that your hands rest at the level of your hipbone—no lower.

> ### DON'T
>
> - Carry anything heavier than your baby for the first two weeks following a vaginal delivery, or for the first month following a cesarean.
> - Remain standing for long periods of time.
> - Push a grocery cart.
> - Vacuum.
> - Make beds.
> - Do anything (even watching television) sitting down when you could do it lying down.

If you plan to carry the baby in a Snugli®, make certain that it is properly adjusted. You should be able to kiss the top of the baby's head. Snuglis® have become somewhat controversial recently because their use can aggravate lower back pain. The baby is often improperly adjusted (babies are carried on their mother's backs in every other culture of the world). Snuglis® are useful, however, when the mother is sitting down and the baby faces out.

Don't carry a baby that is over six months old on your hip. His weight will pull your spine to the side, stressing muscles and ligaments.

Don't forget that a baby also needs to be with its parents between meals. Put him in his bouncer seat, where his back will be better supported than in a car seat, while you cook or take a shower.

Don't bend over to lift your older children (or to tie their shoelaces). To lift a child, kneel on one knee, tighten your pelvic floor and abdominal muscles, breathe out, and then stand up with the child in your arms. When tying a child's shoelaces, either bring the child to your level or kneel down to his.

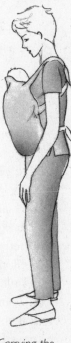

*Carrying the baby in a Snugli®*

### To Carry the Baby Properly
- ✦ Never carry other loads at the same time as you carry the baby.
- ✦ Change the carrying position frequently.

+ Keep up a regular pace when walking.
+ Watch where you put your feet.
+ Don't smoke when you're holding the baby.
+ Hold the baby at chest level, not waist level. Keep her weight well centered. Relax your shoulders.
+ Carry the baby close to your body.
+ Wear comfortable clothes.
+ Wear good quality, comfortable shoes with heels of no more than 1½ inches: 55 percent of our body weight rests on the heels; if your shoe heels are too high, your foot will slide forward and your body will compensate for this imbalance by arching the back, thus causing backache.

Pediatricians recommend that babies be carried with their thighs open 120 degrees. They have to be able to move their legs, stretch and bend their arms, and turn their heads from one side to the other so that they can see everything going on around them.

## In Your Home

### Sitting Down
+ Before sitting, tighten your pelvic floor and abdominal muscles.
+ In a car: Make sure that your knees are at the same level as your pelvis. When you get out of a car, imagine that you are a movie star arriving at a premiere: slide your buttocks to the edge of the seat, pivot your legs out of the car one after the other, push down on the edges of the seat with both hands, and stand up smiling.
+ When breast-feeding: Make certain that your back is well supported and that you are relaxed. Use as many pillows and cushions as necessary to feel comfortable. If your shoulders feel tight or slump forward, the baby is too low. Put a pillow on your knees and place the baby on top of it . . . almost all women need to do this. It is best to have your legs elevated or knees bent at right angles, to help relieve stress on your back and neck.

  Each time you breast-feed, take the time to relax the tension that often builds up in your neck and shoulders: lift your arms above your head, rotate your shoulders, massage your upper back, look up at the ceiling, arch your back, and breathe deeply.

+ Sitting at the computer: Make sure that your feet rest flat on the floor, and that your chair is high enough to allow your chest, shoulders, and upper back to relax.

## In Bed

+ Lying down: Sit on the edge of the bed. Lift both legs off the floor and onto the bed while you pivot on your buttocks. Lie down on your back. Keep your knees bent, and finish by rolling onto your side.

+ Getting up: Don't twist your body or move with your knees apart. First, tighten your abdominal muscles, bend your knees and roll onto your side. Then push yourself up with one hand, slide both legs over the bed with knees together, pivoting on your buttocks, and stand up. Never lead any motion with your neck.

+ Don't ever push up on your elbows—you'll strain your back.

+ While lying down, you should support the full length of your back with pillows—at least two or three in the curve of your back (but no so many as to push your chest forward), and another one behind the shoulders. While lying stretched out on your back, be sure to place a pillow beneath your knees to relieve strain on your lower back.

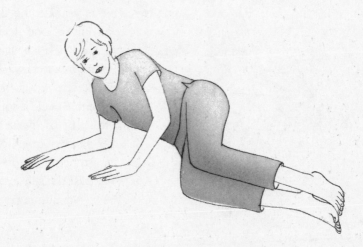

*Lying down*

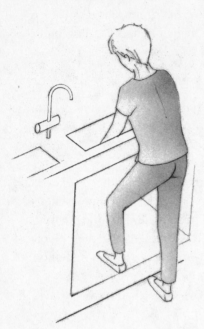

*Doing the dishes*

*Kneel when doing
anything below
waist level*

### Housework

♦ Loading most dishwashers is not recommended during the last months of pregnancy and for the first three months after delivery, unless you kneel down to the floor each time you put a dish in. Ask your partner to do the loading. The next time you remodel a kitchen or install a new dishwasher, remember to have it raised high enough so that you can load and unload it without straining your back.

♦ Washing dishes: Your sink is the right height if you can rest both of your hands flat on its bottom without stooping. If not, wash your dishes in a plastic tub that is raised up to the right level (on top of another inverted tub for example). If your back starts to ache as you do the dishes or cook, raise one foot by resting it on a brick, a thick book, or an inverted washtub.

♦ Always keep your knees slightly bent. Kneel or squat to do anything below waist level, keeping your back as straight as possible (especially when vacuuming).

# Exercises for the First Six Weeks
# After Childbirth

It's practically impossible to keep up a regular exercise program for the first six weeks after childbirth. It's hard enough to remember the nine minutes a day of pelvic floor exercises that we recommend you begin in the first days after childbirth (see pages 79 to 81). But about forty days after giving birth, around the time of their postnatal visit, most women spontaneously feel that they want to get back into shape. This is the point when some outside encouragement—from your ob/gyn, a physical therapist, midwife, or some other specialist in postnatal fitness—really makes a difference.

## Reminder: Two Essential Exercises

As we mentioned earlier, there are two simple, gentle exercises that all new mothers should do during the six weeks after childbirth.

### Restoring Your Pelvic Balance
Lying on your back, legs relaxed, feel the small of your back. Bend your knees; open your legs to hip width, feet flat on the floor. Place your hands on your stomach and feel yourself breathe. Follow the movement of your hands as you breathe in and out: as you inhale, your hands rise and separate; as you exhale, they fall and close together. Then, breathe out as slowly as possible, bringing your stomach in as far as you can without straining. You are stimulating your abdominal muscles by lifting and directing them back to the proper position. Little by little, this will make your belly feel less empty—you are reclaiming your body.

Continue by lightly pressing the soles of your feet against the floor. Gently tighten your buttocks. This puts your pelvis in the proper position: the pubic bone rises, the small of the back flattens, the back stretches out and relaxes, the stomach muscles tighten a bit more, and the pelvic floor is pulled up.

### Pelvic Floor Awareness
Lying on your back on a hard surface, knees bent, focus on your pelvic floor (this exercise is much less efficient when you are standing as your body weight puts three times more pressure on the pelvic floor than when you are lying down).

Try one or more of these possibilities:

◆ Squeeze your anal sphincter as if you were trying to hold back gas. Relax.

◆ Squeeze your urinary sphincter, as if you were trying to stop yourself in the middle of urinating. Relax.

◆ Tighten the walls on the side of your vagina. Relax.

◆ If you manage to stimulate one or more of these muscles, your pelvic floor is being exercised. Concentrate as much on the sensation of relaxing your muscles as on squeezing them.

Don't mistake tightening your abdomen, buttocks, or the inside of your thighs for tightening your pelvic floor. The feeling of pressure on the perineum that is caused by tightening these muscles can be easily be confused with the feeling of tightening the pelvic floor.

By squeezing and relaxing your pelvic floor muscles, you are in fact improving the blood flow to the genital area and accelerating the healing process. You are also restoring a sense of balance to the pelvic region that will help you to overcome the feelings of emptiness and lower body numbness that often follow childbirth.

## A SECRET RECIPE
## AN HOUR'S WALK EACH DAY

About a month after delivery, a great way to resume your normal activity is to walk an hour a day. This will have an amazing effect on your psyche: you'll feel less tired, less depressed, and you'll sleep better. Walking seems to dissolve fatigue—it's a good habit to keep up for the rest of your life. For maximum effect you should follow these rules:

• Don't cheat; do your walking outdoors, for a full hour.
• Wear good shoes.
• Pay attention to your posture, particularly the position of your shoulders and pelvis.
• Walk fast, don't run—no jogging yet.
• If you are not pushing a stroller or baby carriage, swing your arms freely, below chest height.

You should try to do these two exercises three times in the day, repeating the contractions about thirty or forty times. Once your pelvic area no longer feels sore, see if you can hold the contraction for three or four seconds.

## Hygiene

Upon your return from the hospital, you will still be bleeding. If you have had a cesarean or an episiotomy, your scars will not be fully healed for several weeks. The newborn is also quite vulnerable to infections. For all of these reasons, it is important to be particularly careful about your hygiene and the cleanliness of your home (especially your bathroom) during the postnatal period.

- ✦ Make sure that your bathroom is disinfected regularly.
- ✦ Change your washcloth and towel as often as necessary. Use a separate towel to dry your genital area. If you've had an episiotomy or are still raw, use sterile compresses for your personal hygiene.
- ✦ Wash your hands before handling the baby (remind visitors and your other children to do so as well). Remember to wash your hands after changing his diaper. You may want to use a liquid antibacterial soap, which is more hygienic than bar soap.
- ✦ Keep your nails short—a lot of dirt gets trapped under long nails.

## Bleeding

In the first part of this book, you can find a detailed description about how the uterus cleanses and restores itself during the first four weeks after childbirth. For the first four days, the discharge (*lochia*) is blood red but then lightens to a pinkish color. It contains sloughed-off uterine cells and extracellular liquid. Later, the lochia turn to a brownish yellow, then finally to a white discharge. Lochia tend to be more abundant after a cesarean.

Sometimes, the bleeding may suddenly increase or become red again. This usually means that you are being too active. A few days of proper rest should solve the problem. Some women whose bleeding has almost stopped may start bleeding again about twelve days after delivery. This signals the early return of ovarian activity, but not a full return of the menstrual cycle. Other women may notice a temporary return of red bleeding one or two weeks after childbirth, which is due to the sloughing off of the uterine lining at the placental attachment point.

However, bleeding can be the symptom of a more serious problem. If the lochia become bright red or remain scant but appear to drag on, call your doctor or midwife. He/she will probably check for a uterine infection or placental retention (see pages 84 to 89). He/she may advise several days of bed rest and/or a prescription of a synthetic oxytocin, which will help the uterus to contract, and expel any clots or tissue remaining inside.

If lochia become bright red again AND you notice the following symptoms, go to your nearest emergency room or call an ambulance:

+ You completely soak several sanitary pads within a few hours.
+ You pass large clots (the size of golf balls).

You may have a postpartum hemorrhage that is a medical emergency and requires immediate attention.

---

### LATE BLEEDING

**Homeopathy**
- If you are generally weak with cramps and spasms low in your pelvis: Caulophyllum 5C three times a day.
- If you have a random jumble of symptoms, a sense of emotional and physical fragmentation: Cimifuga 5C three times a day.
- If you feel a sense of extreme changeability, emotions close to the surface, and restlessness: Pulsatilla 5C three times a day.
- If you feel strong bearing-down sensations and irritability: Sepia 5C three times a day.
- If you have intermittent bleeding, girdle-like pains and are passing clots: Sabina 30C three times a day.
- China 5C three times a day helps overcome the aftereffects of excessive or prolonged blood loss.

A hemorrhage that occurs one or two weeks after delivery is usually caused by a piece of the placenta that has been retained in the uterus. At the hospital, an ultrasound scan can determine the cause of bleeding, and retained tissue can be removed under anesthesia by curettage.

# Healing your scars

## The Episiotomy Scar

If your episiotomy scar is still painful more than two weeks after childbirth, contact your midwife or doctor. It could be that your stitches have not dissolved properly. The midwife or doctor can remedy this with a simple snip of the annoying stitch. He/she may also prescribe an ointment to speed stitch absorption.

However, if you notice that the episiotomy scar is swollen, red, oozing pus, or extremely tender to the touch, or if you have a fever of more than 100°F. for longer than twenty-four hours, you may have developed an infection. Contact your midwife or doctor immediately. He/she will prescribe an antibiotic therapy or may perform a small local procedure to drain the wound. It's important to treat an episiotomy infection right away because the bacteria may attack your internal stitches before your tissues have healed completely. Even though your skin may be intact on the outside, the tissue inside may remain permanently torn.

## The Cesarean Scar

A cesarean incision usually remains sensitive for about six to eight weeks after surgery. It may itch for up to five months after your delivery. From time to time, it may suddenly become red and itchy before shrinking to its permanent shape, about eight months after the surgery.

In your first few weeks at home, you should be particularly careful about hygiene and follow any instructions for caring for the cesarean scar that you may have received before leaving the hospital. Watch the scar closely for signs of inflammation, such as redness or pus, especially if it is accompanied by a fever of more than 100°F. that lasts for more than twenty-four hours. Contact your doctor or midwife immediately if these symptoms occur.

## HEALING SCAR TISSUE

### The Episiotomy Scar

- Aromatherapy prescribes warm sitz baths for ten to fifteen minutes at a time, in which several drops of essential oil of Calendula or Lavender, and 2 drops essential oil of Cypress have been mixed in the water (Cypress is antiseptic, and Lavender is soothing).
- If you find the cold to be more soothing, apply gauze compresses soaked in a cup of ice-cold water into which 2 drops essential oil of Lavender and 1 drop of essential oil of Chamomile have been added.

### The Cesarean Scar

- Once the scar has healed, massage the area three times a day with Vitamin E oil or Almond oil into which 2 drops essential oil of Siliprele have been added.
- For three or four days in running, apply a poultice of green clay (available in health food stores) to the scar and leave on for two hours.
- Do not expose the scar to direct sun for a year. You may however expose your scar to sunlight coming in through the window for about 10 minutes a day.

### Homeopathy (for both types of scars)

- Take 5 granules Staphysagria 9C morning and evening for ten days; it speeds the healing process.
- Take 5 granules Graphites 15C morning and evening for a month if the scar is painful and swollen.

# Infections

New mothers are vulnerable to infection because their resistance is lower than usual. Good hygiene is the best prevention for urinary and vaginal infections.

## Urinary Infections

Pregnancy and delivery create a number of conditions that increase the risk of developing a urinary infection: more work for the kidneys during pregnancy, bladder distension and compression of the urethra during delivery, irritation from urinary catheters used during a cesarean, and urine retention after delivery. Warning signs for urinary infection include:

+ The urge to urinate frequently, even though little urine comes out.
+ Stinging or burning with urination.
+ Dark, reddish, or murky urine.
+ Abdominal or lower back pain.
+ Fever higher than 100°F. for longer than twenty-four hours, combined with any of above symptoms.

If you notice any of these symptoms, contact your doctor or midwife immediately.

Most doctors will order a urinalysis before prescribing medication. In the meantime, drink a glass of water every hour for ten or twelve hours. Avoid caffeine and all sweet drinks (except unsweetened cranberry juice) as bacteria feed on the sugar in your urine.

## Vaginal Infections

During pregnancy, the sugar levels in the vagina are higher than normal, thus making it more acidic and more vulnerable to infections. The pH of the vagina takes several months to normalize after a delivery. Fatigue also makes women more susceptible to fungal (yeast) infection. The warning signs for a vaginal infection are as follows:

+ Itching, burning, or a white, practically odorless, cheesy discharge. The fungus which causes this type of infection is called *candida albicans*. Reducing your sugar intake helps reduce the acidity of the vagina.

**TIP**

If you are susceptible to yeast infections, cut down on refined sugar during the postnatal period. Eat live-culture yogurt and drink sugar-free cranberry juice (100 percent juice).

◆ Itching and a yellow/green, foamy discharge with a bad smell.
This is probably a parasitic infection.
◆ A foul-smelling discharge without itching could be the sign of
a genital infection, which is producing pus.

Contact your midwife or doctor immediately if you notice any of
these symptoms.

Antibiotics destroy the normal flora (lactobacilli) of the vagina whose
role is to maintain its proper pH balance and to prevent infections. If you
are susceptible to yeast infections, ask for an antifungal treatment (usually a vaginal suppository) whenever you are prescribed antibiotics.

Avoid sexual intercourse when you have a vaginal infection. Your
partner may catch the infection from you, and since men do not always
display symptoms, he may reinfect you without your knowing it. That's
why it's usually recommended that men also be treated.

Wear cotton underpants and avoid wearing tight trousers and
pantyhose. Wash your genital area with pH neutral soap. Do not take
bubble baths.

The stress of the postnatal period can sometimes cause an outbreak
of herpes in women who carry the herpes virus. If you have a herpes
infection, your doctor has probably already advised you of precautions
to take during an outbreak. Be sure to follow these carefully as this is a
dangerous infection for newborns.

In general, avoid taking a bath with your baby if you have any sort
of infection. Put a towel over your knees while you breast-feed to create an additional barrier between the baby and the infected area. Wash
your hands with a disinfectant soap (sold in drugstores) after touching
your genital area. Don't dry your hands on the same towel that you use
to dry the genital area. Always wash the baby's clothes and towels sep-
arately. Don't hand-wash contaminated articles in the same sink or tub
as the one in which you wash your baby's clothes—or else clean the
basin afterwards with chorine bleach.

## Your Appearance

Over two-thirds of women feel uncomfortable about their bodies during the postnatal period. Nevertheless, it is extremely unwise to start a
diet for at least six weeks after childbirth. Here are a few tricks to feel

## YEAST INFECTIONS/THRUSH

### Herbal Remedies
- Drink an infusion of Echinacea, Cleavers, and Chamomile three times a day.
- If you feel a burning sensation, compresses of an infusion of Marigold, Chamomile, American Cranesbill, Beth Root, Echinacea, Cleavers, and Wild Indigo are very soothing.
- It is recommended that you eat plenty of garlic, cabbage, raw kale, and turnips.

### Aromatherapy
Use 5 drops essential oil of Tea Tree in a bath. Compresses dipped in a solution of boiled water and 2 percent Tea Tree essential oil may also help. Add essential oil of Lavender or Chamomile to water to make a soothing vulval wash.

Also make sure that you are getting enough of the following vitamins and minerals: A, B-complex, C, zinc, iron and magnesium. Take probiotics, acidophilous and bifidobacteria (generally added to certain yogurts).

a little less demoralized about excess weight, a sagging stomach, flabby muscles, lackluster hair, and a tired complexion:

Use a pretty camisole or slip to hide your maternity bra and your big stomach.

Most maternity clothes will not fit properly within a few days after childbirth, yet very few women are able to wear their pre-pregnancy clothes for many weeks to come. But don't succumb to buying a whole new wardrobe two sizes bigger than your normal size! Being able to wear your "normal" clothes once again is one of the best incentives to getting your figure back. In the meantime, satisfy your urge for a make-over with accessories and a few inexpensive items that can tide you over the coming weeks—a large shirt or sweater over leggings is particularly comfortable.

Blouses and dresses that button down the front are more practical for nursing than T-shirts or pullovers, which tend to fall over the baby's face and leave the breasts uncovered.

Beware of delicate fabrics—breast milk and spit up can ruin them forever (soda water works wonders to deodorize regurgitated milk).

Don't be surprised if your feet grow a half size bigger after your first delivery. (Fortunately it only happens once!)

Try the "look good, feel good" approach: use makeup or wear accessories that make you feel attractive and improve your attitude about your appearance.

## Hair and Skin

Pregnant women are known to have a radiant complexion. The texture of the skin is oilier and pregnant women perspire more, but their skin is moister and suppler. Nails, hair, and skin cells grow faster. Women who are prone to acne see a distinct improvement in their condition during the second two trimesters of pregnancy. Elevated hormone levels of pregnancy cause these changes. After childbirth, the drop in hormone levels unfortunately has the opposite effect, often aggravated by the fatigue and anemia that are so common after delivery. The skin usually becomes normal again once the menstrual cycle returns. But acne-prone women find that their skin breaks out for several weeks or months after childbirth. This may be due not only to fluctuating hormone levels but also to stress, a major cause of acne in adults.

Supplementing your zinc intake (found in green vegetables—spinach, watercress, and broccoli—whole grains, beans, mushrooms, brewer's yeast, seafood, and meat) can be helpful to your hair and skin.

Pregnancy hormones cause pigmentation zones on the breasts and external genitalia, both of which will probably remain a darker color after your first pregnancy. The stretching of skin tissues in the belly area may cause a vertical brown line (*linea nigra*) to appear between your umbilicus and your pubis. It usually will disappear about three months after childbirth. In the meantime, don't expose your stomach to the sun. Some women, especially brunettes, get a "pregnancy mask," also known as *chloasma* (brownish spots that appear most often on the forehead, temples, and cheeks). Since these spots will intensify if exposed to the sun, women are advised to wear strong sunblock throughout their pregnancy and for several months after childbirth (a pregnancy mask generally disappears within three months after childbirth but can persist for up to one year, especially if the woman takes oral contraceptives). Don't hesitate to see a dermatologist if the mask remains visible for more than three months, and avoid direct sun exposure.

## YOUR SKIN AFTER PREGNANCY

The following aromatherapy remedies can be used to massage your skin, particularly your belly and thighs.

Mix:

- 2 drops essential oil of Geranium
- 10 drops essential oil of Lavender
- 5 drops essential oil of Ylang-Ylang
- 8 drops essential oil of Sandalwood
  in 50 ml milliliters base oil.

Or for a smaller quantity, mix:

- 1 drop essential oil of Geranium
- 2 drops essential oil of Lavender
- 1 drop essential oil of Ylang-Ylang
- 1 drop essential oil of Sandalwood
  in 2 tablespoons of base oil.

- Blue Orchid or Sandalwood oil can also be used.
- Evening Primrose oil (available in capsules), an excellent hormonal regulator, is effective against dryness due to lower hormone levels.
- Calendula cream, Echinacea, or Evening Primrose oil all help to lighten pigmentation spots.

You should also watch carefully for new moles. During pregnancy, precancerous changes in moles develop four times as fast. Don't wait until you have had your baby to consult a dermatologist if you notice any of the following signs:

- ✦ Appearance of new moles that are black.
- ✦ Change in any existing moles (in color, size, and width).
- ✦ A mole with unusual coloration (blue, gray, pink) or with an uneven shape.

Even if you have your baby in winter, avoid sun exposure the following summer so those pigmentation spots will not reappear. Most importantly, avoid perspiring or using perfumed beauty products in the sun, as their acidity darkens pigmentation.

Vascular red spots called *star angiomas*, and blood moles on the trunk (*cherry angiomas*) may also appear during pregnancy. They will disappear by themselves, or can be burned off by a dermatologist. If you already have skin tags (*fibroepithelial polyps*), they may grow even bigger.

Some women get their first bout of *perioral dermatitis* (ugly red rash around the mouth and chin which resembles acne) during pregnancy. The only cure is a course of oral tetracycline, which must wait until after the baby is weaned (acne medication will make it worse). The skin may still be prone to flare-ups for six months to two years.

## Stretch Marks

During pregnancy, the skin over the belly, breasts, hips, and thighs can be stretched to the point that its fibers tear. These weakened areas show up as purple or reddish marks that can be up to half an inch wide. Stretch marks are most obvious during the weeks after delivery, but in most cases, they gradually narrow to fine white lines. Sometimes, however, stretch marks can remain unsightly and annoying; a lot depends on the initial elasticity of your skin before pregnancy. Added to the problem of stretch marks is the fact that the stretched skin of the breasts and stomach may have trouble shrinking back after delivery. There exist several possible treatments if stretch marks remain highly visible six months after delivery:

- Dermabrasion, which peels off the top layers of the epidermis, can lighten stretch marks. But results vary from one woman to another. Beware of poorly trained practitioners.
- A French study has found Vitamin A acid cream (Retin-A, used in treating acne), which can be prescribed by a dermatologist, to be helpful especially when used right after childbirth (never during pregnancy) when the marks are still pink and fresh. Its use must be supervised carefully.
- Laser therapy and cryotherapy (freezing) often do more harm than good.

+ For stretch marks which are at least ¼ inch wide, plastic surgery can pull together the stretched skin and sew together the
  edges of healthy skin. A thin linear scar will remain.
+ Liposuction of the abdomen does not make stretch marks disappear but those appearing on excess skin will be removed.

Whatever treatment you choose, it's important to never massage
skin that has heavy stretch marks, regardless of whether you use cream
or not.


## Hair

The hormonal changes of pregnancy can have all sorts of effects on
hair: it can change color, become shinier or duller. Curly hair can
become straight, and straight hair can become curly.

Normally, a woman loses about a hundred hairs a day. During the
nine months of pregnancy, high hormone levels keep hair from falling
out and estrogen gives hair a shinier and silkier appearance and keeps
the ends from splitting. But the hair that has been retained during pregnancy has to fall out some day. Between the third and sixth month after
childbirth (often when weaning takes place or when the baby begins to

---

### YOUR HAIR AFTER PREGNANCY

**Herbal Remedies**

• Mix dried herbs of Bardane, Nettle, Serpolet, and Thyme in equal quantities. Throw a handful into a quart of boiling water and let it boil for fifteen
  minutes. Once cooled, apply to your hair. Cover your head with a shower
  cap and a hot towel for one hour, and then rinse. This treatment nour-
  ishes the capillaries and helps restore your hair's body and shine.

• Ground Linseed, about ¼ cup a day, eaten mixed in salad or vegetables
  can improve hair quality.

• Copper supplements are helpful if your hair is lifeless and lacks body after
  childbirth. This mineral also can be found in oysters, dried fruits, whole
  grains, almonds, dried pulses, green vegetables, fresh fruit (particularly red
  and black currants, blackberries, apples, and pears). Zinc and vitamin $B_6$
  supplements are also effective.

eat solids), most women feel like they are losing great handfuls of hair each day (the peak is generally at six months).

Some women notice the appearance of more facial hair during pregnancy. This is also caused by hormonal changes.

Many hairdressers advise that just after delivery hair should be cut and principally air dried, and then brushed well morning and evening to eliminate dead cells and improve scalp circulation.

Copper is especially recommended for hair. It's found in oysters, grains, dried fruits, almonds, broad beans (lima and fava), green vegetables, and fresh fruit (especially currants, apples, and pears). Zinc and vitamin $B_6$ are also helpful. Be sure to reduce your alcohol and coffee consumption (if you are not breast-feeding—if you are, you probably should not be taking coffee or alcoholic beverages anyway), as they both tend to deplete your ability to store the B vitamins, which are essential for good hair quality.

You may also notice that your nails chip more easily or have white spots. This is a sign that you need to supplement your mineral intake. It helps to massage your nails with almond oil.

## Teeth and Gums

It used to be said that a woman lost a tooth with each pregnancy. It is indeed true that the impact of pregnancy hormones (especially progesterone) on the microcirculation of the mouth leads to gum inflammation. This also explains why some pregnant women have frequent nosebleeds. "Pregnancy gingivitis," which affects up to 60 percent of all pregnant women, causes the gums to become tender, red, and to bleed easily, sometimes profusely. Plaque forms more rapidly. In some extreme cases (5 percent of the time) a "pregnancy tumor" (*epulis*) forms. This is a growth on the gum that can be as big as an inch and may cover a tooth. Since it will bleed easily, it must be excised during pregnancy (or if it is little, it may disappear spontaneously after childbirth).

Dental problems affect one-third of all pregnant women; they start in about the second month of pregnancy, and may worsen in about the eighth month. An inflammation of the gums already present before pregnancy may worsen. After childbirth, the gums will return to the condition they were in at the second month of pregnancy. A grayish line may appear at the base of the bottom teeth. Untreated, the gums will take some time to return to their normal condition. Relapses are common and the problem usually will recur in the following pregnancy. Furthermore, pregnancy uses up the body's calcium stores, and teeth are more vulnerable to cavities during this period. These are all reasons to see a dentist regularly both during pregnancy and soon after childbirth.

A pregnant woman should pay special attention to her dental hygiene, brushing her teeth three times a day and rinsing her mouth. At the beginning of her pregnancy she should visit the dentist to have her teeth cleaned, and then again in the fourth, eighth, and tenth months.

Soon after delivery (when you have enough energy), make an appointment with your dentist for a thorough cleaning to get rid of plaque and tartar.

After your menstrual cycle resumes, it's time to get rid of any "periodontal pockets" (little sacks of gum tissue that harbor bacteria) that have appeared or worsened during pregnancy. If these pockets are not eliminated, there is a large risk of relapse of gingivitis in spite of careful cleaning. If this procedure requires a local anesthesia, there is no risk to a breast-feeding baby. Afterwards, you can return to a routine schedule of twice yearly dental checkups.

In addition to dental care, you can supplement your calcium and phosphorus intake (available in green vegetables, grains, dried fruit, milk, and cheese).

## Eyes

The shape of the eyeball often changes during pregnancy (which explains why most optometrists will not fit a new pair of contacts on a pregnant woman). It will be back to its pre-pregnant state about six to nine months after birth. The hormonal changes of pregnancy may also temporarily alter the shape of the cornea.

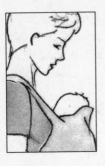

# 10

# Diet After Childbirth

During her pregnancy, a woman pays special attention to her health. She goes for monthly medical checkups, watches her diet and weight, avoids pollutants and contact with toxic substances, rests more often, tries to exercise in moderation and spend more time outdoors. So, why not keep these good habits? As we state throughout this book, a woman's body is more vulnerable during the postnatal period. It takes a special effort to get it back into shape. Proper nutrition is an essential part of this process.

## The Impact of Childbirth

Pregnancy and delivery diminish the body's nutritional reserves. For nine months the pregnant woman's body provides all that is needed to manufacture another human being. She then loses about 400 ml of blood during her delivery and almost 100 ml more in the weeks that follow. The childbirth uses up the body's reserves of vitamins, mineral salts, and trace elements. Finally, the recovery process, which includes mending any damage that may have occurred during delivery, creates

| Non–breast-feeding Mothers | | Breast-feeding Mothers | |
|---|---|---|---|
| Calories | 2,000 | Calories | 2,500 |
| Protein | 70 g | Protein | 80 g |
| Carbohydrates | 275 g | Carbohydrates | 275 to 350 g |
| Alphanoleic acid | 3.5 to 4.5 g | Alphanoleic acid | 3.5 to 4.5 g |
| Iron | 18 to 25 mg* | Iron | 13 mg |
| Calcium | 1,200 to 1,500 mg | Calcium | 1,200 to 1,500 mg |
| Phosphorus | 1,000 mg | Phosphorus | 1,000 mg |
| Magnesium | 480 mg | Magnesium | 480 mg |
| Zinc | 15 mg | Zinc | 19 mg |
| Copper | 3 mg | Copper | 3 mg |
| Iodine | 175 mcg | Iodine | 200 mcg |
| Selenium | 65 mcg | Selenium | 75 mcg |
| Vitamin A | 1,000 mcg | Vitamin A | 1,300 mcg |
| Vitamin D | 20 mcg | Vitamin D | 15 mcg |
| Vitamins $B_1$ and $B_2$ | 1.8 mg | Vitamins $B_1$ and $B_2$ | 1.8 mg |
| Vitamin $B_6$ | 2.5 mg | Vitamin $B_6$ | 2.5 mg |
| Folic Acid | 800 mcg | Folic Acid | 800 mcg |
| Vitamin $B_{12}$ | 4 mcg | Vitamin $B_{12}$ | 4 mcg |
| Viamin E | 20 mg | Vitamin E | 20 mg |
| Vitamin C | 90 mg | Vitamin C | 90 mg |

*Women who don't breast-feed require more iron because they generally start menstruating six to eight weeks after delivery.

extra nutritional needs. In short, the postnatal period is the time to cor-rect imbalances and replenish stocks. Here are the nutritional require-ments the first three months after delivery.

## How to Get What You Need

Keep taking the prenatal vitamins prescribed during pregnancy for at least three months postpartum, longer if you continue breast-feeding. Too many women stop taking their vitamins after delivery.

Eat fresh foods—naturopaths recommend consuming more raw, untreated food than normal (lots of salads and raw vegetables). Now is the time to spend a little more money on organic foods. Also, remem-ber that the way in which you cook food will determine how many vitamins are left by the time it reaches your plate.

Take supplementary minerals if necessary. Less well known than vitamins, minerals and trace elements are metals and metalloids that are necessary for many of the body's biochemical reactions. Deficiency of a trace element can lead to a slowing of some of the body's vital mechanisms such as the immune system, oxygen transport, or digestion.

Mothers who are vegetarians can certainly maintain a diet to support their nutritional needs. But since vitamin $B_{12}$ is found only in the animal kingdom, deficiencies may occur when a mother maintains a "vegan" diet, excluding eggs and milk products as well as meat. Supplementation with up to 4 mg of vitamin $B_{12}$ per day is recommended.

## Special Needs During the Postpartum Period

### Iron

The normal hemoglobin level of a woman in good health is from 12 to 14 g per 100 ml of blood. It allows for the production of the red pigment that transports oxygen to all parts of the body. If the iron level drops below 10 g per 100 ml of blood, anemia sets in. When menstruating, a woman loses a total of 30 ml of blood a month, which is the equivalent of 0.5 mg iron. Therefore, it is easy to understand that the blood loss of delivery, and then of lochia, can have an impact on hemoglobin levels. A woman is said to be anemic when her level of red blood cells falls below a certain point. If a woman already is anemic at the end of her pregnancy (30 percent of all women begin their pregnancy with an iron deficiency; 70 percent finish pregnancy with iron stores that are almost totally depleted), the problem can worsen with the slowdown in circulation that occurs after childbirth. Anemia can also appear in women who had normal hemoglobin levels before delivery. This is why most doctors systematically continue to prescribe iron after childbirth. A new mother needs a supplement of 2.5 mg per day. It takes at least three months to replenish iron reserves.

An anemic woman is tired, listless, and depressed. She may have palpitations of the heart, tingling, or numbness of the extremities, or she may feel cold much of the time. Anemia can also cause digestive problems such as nausea, gas, abdominal distention, diarrhea, or constipation. Two dietary strategies can help to rebuild iron stores:

First, eat an iron-rich diet, with iron from animal sources (meat and fish) and vegetable sources (spinach, lentils, avocados, oats, wheat germ, brewer's yeast, dried beans, and peas), as well as certain seaweeds like Carlton (available in health food stores), dried fruit, and nuts.

Iron from animal sources is more available for use by the human body, because it takes a form that is more readily absorbed than iron from plant sources; we are able to retain 15 percent of it, as opposed to 5 percent of the iron in vegetables.

It is important to remember that iron must work with other nutrients in the body to increase red blood cell production. For example, iron from plant sources needs vitamin C in order to be absorbed, so citrus fruits (orange, lemon, and grapefruit) and other foods rich in vitamin C should be eaten regularly to maximize iron absorption. In fact, anemia can be due not to an iron deficiency but to insufficient vitamin $B_{12}$ or folic acid or manganese or copper or vitamin $B_6$—all necessary for iron absorption by the body.

*A tip:* Sprouts are extremely rich in iron and calcium.

Another strategy is to consume trace elements that facilitate the absorption of iron by the body: copper, zinc (which is necessary for more than 100 of the body's biochemical reactions to occur), molybdenum, manganese (active in hormonal and neurologic processes), cobalt, and selenium.

*Caution:* Tannins in black tea bind to iron and will eliminate it in urine. Therefore a new mother should not drink more than two cups of tea per day.

## Proteins

Normally a woman needs about ½ g protein per pound per day. In the postnatal period she needs 5 extra g per day to repair tissues damaged in delivery, and an additional 5 g if she is breast-feeding.

The consumption of animal protein is controversial. Meat contains complete proteins, in large concentrations (20 percent) which allows women to consume a smaller quantity in order to meet their protein needs. Fish is 15 to 20 percent protein. On the other hand, certain plant protein sources—like soy flour (37 percent), lentils (24 percent), and beans (18 percent)—contain practically as much "incomplete" protein as meat and fish, as well as complex carbohydrates and fiber. They do, however, need to be completed with grains and other complementary proteins to be useful.

## Calcium

To build a baby's skeleton, a mother uses 150 g per day from her own calcium stores. Calcium is the most abundant mineral in the body, the essential element of the cellular membrane; it allows the release of many hormones, the coagulation of blood, and the contraction of muscle fiber. Normally a woman needs 900 mg calcium per day; a pregnant woman needs 1,300 mg, and a new mother needs 1,600 mg for as long as she is breast-feeding. Symptoms of calcium deficiency include muscle cramps and depression.

Dairy products provide two-thirds of our daily calcium needs. Don't forget that low-fat and skim milk have as much calcium and B vitamins as whole milk. Parmesan is the cheese with the highest calcium content. The calcium content of an eight-ounce glass of milk is the equivalent of two eight-ounce yogurts or of an ounce of Swiss cheese.

Fortunately for women who are lactose intolerant, vegan, or who are suffering from severe hemorrhoids, dairy products are not the only source of calcium: supplements are widely available in pill form, as well as certain brands of mineral water, calcium-fortified orange juice, almonds, tahini (chickpea paste), tofu, watercress, sprouts (100 g bean sprouts have 71 mg calcium), and broccoli.

It is also important to consume a calcium/magnesium ratio of 2/1 (see below) and a calcium/phosphorus ratio of 1/1 (the ratio usually found in food) for both of these minerals to be absorbed properly.

Vitamin D, which is produced by the skin from sunlight, is stored in the calcium of tooth and bone cells.

## Magnesium

While calcium makes muscles contract, magnesium makes them relax. It is the mineral that has the greatest effect on the nervous system, and on mood. A magnesium deficiency makes one more vulnerable to stress. People with magnesium deficiencies will have these symptoms: nervousness, fatigue, tight throat (difficulty breathing), dizziness, headaches, itching, restless sleep, decreased libido, and depression.

Unfortunately, the good dietary sources of magnesium are often high in calories: dried beans and split peas, shrimp, bran, whole grains, dried fruit and nuts, cocoa and chocolate, as well as snails, periwinkles, and clams. But you can buy supplements as well as drink mineral water that is high in magnesium content (a trace element that is particularly well absorbed when it comes from an aqueous source). Be care-

## TO SUMMARIZE

In addition to protein, dairy products, fruits and vegetables, as discussed above, the daily diet of a woman during the postnatal period should include:

- Liver or fatty fish, three times a week
- Three pieces of fruit and two fresh vegetables per day
- Two tablespoons of oil in a salad or with raw vegetables
- Whole grain bread
- Mineral water that is high in calcium
- Ten nuts (almonds, walnuts, or hazelnuts)
- Eight glasses of mineral water (preferably with a high calcium content)

ful, though: in large doses, magnesium is a strong laxative. Intake, therefore, should be spread out over three meals. Calcium and magnesium need to coexist in the body's cells in order to be effective.

### Fiber

Fiber is necessary to assure the transit of food through the intestinal system. During pregnancy, intestinal muscle capacity is reduced and is not fully restored until two or three months after childbirth due to the continued presence of pregnancy hormones in the body. Fibers also help eliminate toxins from the body (such as the chemical byproduct of stress: adrenaline).

Fiber needs plenty of water in order to work well. That's one of the reasons that it is necessary to drink enough (eight glasses of water a day) after delivery: hydration is necessary for intestinal transit.

*Beware:* Laxatives with a paraffin base, which are often distributed in hospitals, will bind fat-soluble vitamins (A, D, E, and K) and eliminate them from the body.

## Your Dietary Habits

### Fats

If you change only one thing in your dietary habits, change the fats you consume.

For cooking, replace animal fats with nonhydrogenated vegetable oils (if possible, organic). Animals store toxins in their fat. Naturopaths claim that if our liver uses all of its resources to fight against toxins, it will be less available to use the amino acids needed to rebuild our cells. And for a new mother, cellular renovation is very important.

For salad dressings, use oil from the first, cold press. A good mix for salad dressing is one part olive oil, one part sunflower oil, and one part wheat germ or grapeseed oil.

## Sugar

Watch your sugar intake. Replace refined sugar with honey, dried fruit, or maple syrup.

Avoid the cheapest brands of sweets. Unfortunately, the ingredients found in low-cost foods generally are not of the best quality. Cheap cookies, for example, have more sugar and saturated fat, and artificial rather than real flavorings (vanillin, for example, instead of pure vanilla extract).

If we mention sugar, we should also mention the salt that many new mothers crave. Remember that salt increases the feeling of hunger. Remember also that only about 6 percent of the salt we consume comes from the shaker—the rest is in the canned, bottled, processed, and frozen food we eat . . . another reason for new mothers to eat as much fresh food as possible.

## Vitamin Supplements

Don't load yourself with vitamin supplements: It serves no purpose to absorb quantities that far exceed those found naturally in food. Vitamin pills are no substitute for a balanced diet. The body absorbs natural vitamins better than synthetic ones. Naturopaths claim that synthetic vitamins lack a "vital energy," and therefore don't bind as well in the body.

*Helpful hints:* Blackcurrant seeds, Evening Primrose, and Borage contain gamma-linoleic acid, a fatty acid that is essential to prostaglandin function. They help rebuild the immune system, soften the skin, and above all, smoothly reestablish the ovarian cycle.

## A Word About Dieting

When you return home, it is perfectly normal to still have five or ten pounds (or more!) to lose—they are your body's reserves for breast-feeding. And prolactin, the hormone that regulates milk production, has a tendency to cause water retention. The big belly and thighs of a new mother represent the natural reserves that have allowed the survival of the species. During pregnancy, the surface absorption of the digestive tract increases from 30 to 50 percent. Nutrients are better digested, and in larger quantities, which explains why pregnant women are hungry more often. It will take several months for the digestive tract to return to its normal volume. It is useless to start a diet before then.

Some women think that breast-feeding helps them lose weight; others find that they only lose their last extra pounds after they stop nursing. Women who are still breast-feeding six weeks after delivery lose an average of over two pounds more than women who have stopped by ten days do. **The only time that a woman uses up the fat on her hips is during the time that she breast-feeds**—if she nurses her baby for more than three months. This fat is practically impossible to lose through a typical diet or even exercise.

**To state it bluntly, dieting within the first three months after childbirth is likely to lead to fatigue and failure.** During pregnancy and immediately after childbirth, the body is extremely efficient at storing energy as fat. It takes time for the enzyme involved in this process (lipoprotein lipase) to diminish. The thyroid, which regulates the body's metabolism, slows. As a result, the body will need fewer calories to function and balances energy (calorie) supplies in order to heal itself. The hormonal excesses or deficiencies which often occur in the postnatal period can alter hunger and satiety signals (as a rule, estrogen decreases hunger and progesterone increases it).

Furthermore, weight is controlled by the brain (in the *hypothalamus*). All aspects of daily life (emotional, professional, familial, sociocultural, age) have an impact on the nervous system: weight regulation is influenced by all of our surroundings. The arrival of a new baby is an enormous upheaval. Fatigue, lack of sleep, possible dietary deficiency or anemia, discomfort from incisions or lacerations, and back pain all create poor conditions for weight loss.

Most doctors and midwives recommend that new mothers wait until menstruation returns before starting a serious diet. But if you have let yourself go during the last months of pregnancy, there's no harm in trying to get back on track with good dietary habits. Simply avoiding too much sugar and fat will lead to weight loss!

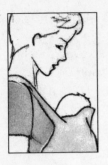

# 11

## Resuming Your Menstrual Cycle

### Your First Period After Childbirth

For a woman who is not breast-feeding, the first period after child-birth often signals that "things are getting back to normal." It occurs six to eight weeks postpartum. If milk production has been blocked by medication, the ovarian cycle will resume even earlier. The first period after childbirth is often heavier and lasts longer than usual, possibly as long as eight days. Some women find that they no longer have menstrual cramps after giving birth (but others claim that there is no change). Sometimes menstrual patterns change for good.

### Your Fertility

You only need to look at the number of families where there is only eleven to thirteen months' difference between children to realize that many women do not fully understand the issue of fertility in the weeks after childbirth. A woman who does not use birth control has a 90 per-cent chance of conceiving in the first year after childbirth.

---

## YOUR FIRST MENSTRUAL CYCLE
## AFTER CHILDBIRTH

### Homeopathy

• Take China 5C if blood loss is very heavy during your first period.

### Herbal Remedies

• A cup of Sage tea after each meal prepared in the following way: 20 g dried leaves per quart of boiling water. Sage is an excellent normalizer of the reproductive system.
• Evening Primrose oil, taken orally in a capsule or in drops of essential oil on a lump of sugar, is a wonderful hormonal regulator and stimulator of ovarian activity.

---

## Basic Principles

Ninety percent of all women will not ovulate before their first period: it will be an anovulatory period, like the period of a woman who is on the pill. There is no way to determine when you will begin to ovulate. (Ten percent of women can ovulate within twenty-one days after giving birth.)

Sperm can survive in the genital tract for five days. For those women who choose to have sexual intercourse so soon after childbirth, contraception must be used from the sixteenth day postpartum.

**Breast-feeding is not a form of contraception**. It is the sensation of the baby sucking that sends a message to the brain to suppress the hormone that stimulates ovulation. The effectiveness of this suppression depends on the strength and frequency of the sucking. For breast-feeding to work as a means of contraception, the baby must nurse full-time, around the clock. That means neither expressing milk nor giving supplementary bottles. If the baby sucks his thumb or a pacifier, this may be enough to diminish the intensity of his sucking. Even a baby who cries a lot also may be too weak to suck with sufficient strength to affect hormonal production by the brain.

Many women only get their period back once they stop breast-feeding. The rest find that their menstrual cycle may resume at any time from about two months after childbirth.

## Contraception

Until your menstrual period returns, many common contraceptive methods are contraindicated or even impossible to use.

**An IUD** cannot be inserted before the menstrual cycle is reestablished. Some physicians require a six-week wait while the uterus is healing and recovering its shape and tone. Introducing a foreign body into a uterus that is still soft and dilated can lead to a serious infection, perforate the walls, or simply be rejected. The pain involved in these complications is not inconsequential.

Most women who use a **diaphragm** as contraception find that their pre-pregnancy diaphragm is now too small. Furthermore, in the weeks after childbirth, the vagina is enlarged and the perineal muscles are lax, which means that a diaphragm cannot act as a proper barrier. For these reasons, the diaphragm must be refitted during your postpartum visit. Only then does it become an effective option.

All the **natural contraceptive methods** (basal body temperature, cervical mucus) are impossible to use because you cannot predict your first ovulation, on which subsequent calculations are based. The enormous changes in hormone levels of pregnancy and the postpartum period also affect the cervical mucus. The vagina is generally quite dry in the weeks following childbirth.

The classic **"combined" estrogen/progesterone pill** is not generally prescribed after delivery because its use at this time has been shown to cause blood clots in the veins and may inhibit milk production.

However, two reliable methods of contraception are recommended: **barrier contraceptives** (such as condoms and spermicides) and the **progesterone mini-pill**.

**Condoms** are the method of choice, unless the walls of the vagina are still very sensitive. In that case, it's better to wait a while longer to have sex. It's important that the penis be withdrawn from the vagina before it has become completely flaccid, so that the condom stays on. (Be careful: some lubricants dissolve latex!)

**Spermicides** are 98 percent effective if they are used correctly. If the bleeding has stopped and the perineum has healed, they can be used as early as twenty days after delivery. The spermicide must cover the entire vaginal wall, so that it forms a barrier to the uterus and can effectively destroy sperm cells. Spermicides exist in the form of vaginal suppositories, foams, and creams, which are inserted with applicators.

It's important to read the instructions before use. Suppositories must be inserted at least five minutes before having intercourse but they are effective for two to twenty-four hours, depending on the brand. However, they can kill only the sperm of one ejaculation. Creams have a contraceptive effect, which generally lasts about ten hours, but also cover only one ejaculation.

**The mini-pill.** This oral contraceptive contains low doses of progesterone, which hinder the production of cervical mucus and thin uterine mucus—much like the combined estrogen/progesterone pill. Ovulation can occur but the uterine lining will not be receptive to implantation of the egg. This pill has a failure rate of between 1 to 3 percent, as well as an increased risk of an ectopic pregnancy if conception does occur. The mini-pill is not contraindicated for breast-feeding, and can be prescribed from the fifteenth day after childbirth (some doctors prescribe it on the fifth day postpartum if a woman is not breast-feeding). The mini-pill must be taken every day at exactly the same time: even taking it three hours late can decrease its effectiveness and cause bleeding. Many women also complain of breakthrough bleeding between periods, caused by the atrophy of the uterine lining. As a result, few women choose to continue this contraceptive method once they wean their baby.

Some women who are at risk for another pregnancy choose to use an injectable contraceptive such as Depo-Provera that lasts from one to three months.

## The Postnatal Visit

For many of the world's major religions, the forty days that follow childbirth are a period of special care and rest, during which the new mother is considered impure. The postnatal visit, which usually takes place about six weeks after childbirth, still symbolically marks the end of the postpartum period.

Nevertheless, many minor ailments persist well after these six weeks. For example, 40 percent of all cases of postnatal depression appear more than forty days after childbirth. So always remember that there is no reason not to contact your doctor or midwife with questions and concerns relating to your pregnancy or delivery even after the postnatal visit has occurred.

## A FEW WORDS OF ADVICE

As with your antenatal visits, you will probably have many questions. Write them down, and then take the time to ask them. If you aren't satisfied with the answers, ask to be referred to a specialist. Don't accept simple reassurances when you are convinced that you have a physical problem. But remember, an obstetrician is not a psychotherapist. If you feel the need to talk about psychological problems, ask your doctor to recommend a specialist in the area. All good doctors have a network of colleagues whom they can recommend.

What happens during the postnatal visit?

+ A urine sample will be taken for analysis.
+ Your blood pressure will be checked.
+ Your weight will be checked.
+ Your abdominal wall will be examined (if you had a cesarean).
+ Your breasts will be examined.
+ You will probably receive an internal exam to check your uterus, cervix, ovaries, and fallopian tubes, as well as the state of your perineum.
+ A Pap smear will be taken if there was a lesion present after delivery. If not, this test will be performed about two months later.
+ Your legs will be examined for swelling and varicose veins.
+ If you are feeling tired, blood may be drawn to check for anemia.
+ Your doctor will discuss your contraception needs with you and refit your diaphragm, if necessary.

The doctor or midwife should then ask you about your emotional state, your diet, your sex life, your relationship with your partner, how you've organized your household, and your professional plans and arrangements for child care.

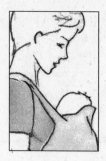

# 12

## Returning
## to Work

Since passage of the Family and Medical Leave Act in 1993 American workers have been entitled to twelve weeks of unpaid maternity leave after the birth of a child. For many women, the decision to return to work is based purely on economics, and going without income for twelve weeks is not possible. For others, their decision is not based on finances alone but on the desire to remain active professionally and to find sources of fulfillment outside the home. In fact, many women feel that their time at work is less stressful—because it is more structured—than their family life!

Numerous studies demonstrate that children will not suffer if their mother's job satisfaction is high. Indeed, working mothers are less prone to depression. Contrary to conventional thinking, mothers have always worked. Since the dawn of time, rural women, factory workers, and those employed in domestic work did not have the luxury to question the psychological impact of their work on their family. Even middle-class women who remained at home were absorbed by domestic chores far more burdensome than those we face today. Until the advent of free and compulsory primary education, children were put to work as soon as possible in order to supplement the family's income—

this is still the case in developing countries. The notion that a "good mother" should stay home rather than have her children raised by someone else is a fairly recent concept. Today it seems that the pendulum has swung the other way: work and child rearing are perceived as two contradictory tasks that are difficult, if not impossible, to accomplish simultaneously. As a result, many women feel demoralized and extremely guilty when returning to work after having a baby. Yet it is not the fact that their mother is working which harms children, it is her feeling of guilt which destabilizes the family. A child is not born with preconceived ideas about whether her mother should work or not. He or she takes life as you offer it: whether you live in the country or the city, whether you are rich or poor. But a child does have an incredible ability to sense the emotions of the parents, especially their feelings of guilt or anguish.

Children do not suffer from being cared for by a person other than their mother. In fact, this can be an enriching experience as long as they feel secure and receive sufficient affection and stimulation. Child psychologists have demonstrated that children blossom when in contact with other children and learn a lot through play. Nevertheless, children are vulnerable to the carelessness of those in whose care they are entrusted. For this reason, it is important to give yourself ample time—early in your pregnancy—to carefully investigate your child-care options, whether a day-care center, home day care, au pair care or family caregivers. This takes time and effort. Once that decision is made, finding the appropriate caregiver is another time-consuming endeavor. But the effort is well worthwhile and should be viewed as an investment in your career as well as in your peace of mind.

**Whatever the reasons for returning to work, preparation early in pregnancy is critical.**

+ No matter how much preparation has been made beforehand no one is fully prepared for the emotional upheaval that occurs even for the most committed professional. Turning the care of your precious newborn over to another can be a heart-wrenching experience. It is important (and often required by day-care centers) to provide a gradual transition to a day-care provider. Start with a few hours a day while you are still at home. In this way, both you and your baby will be able to adjust. Most important is the relationship you develop with your child's caregiver. It is central to your success at work and your child's development. You may wish to use your last day of maternity leave to pay a surprise visit to the day-care center or caregiver to ensure that everything is satisfactory.

+ Explain to your baby that you will be leaving him during the day and when you will be back. Even a tiny baby will be sensitive to the tone of your voice. You may want to leave with him an article of clothing which smells of you.

+ If you have an office job, you may find it helpful to bring yourself "up to speed" while still at home by reading through the most important files which will be waiting for you upon your return.

+ A cell phone or beeper will help you feel more "in touch."

+ It is quite normal for you to be particularly irritable about three days before you start work again. And this may also reflect on the baby, who will feel your anxiety and become fussier as a result.

## Breast-feeding for the Working Mother

Returning to work does not mean that you need to stop breast-feeding. The American Academy of Pediatrics recommends that mothers nurse for at least one year. Unfortunately, only 21 percent of mothers who are employed full-time are still nursing when their baby is six months old (two-thirds of women nurse in the days following the baby's birth). Once a good milk supply has been established, it is possible to empty your breasts by pumping during the hours when you are not with your baby. Emptying your breasts is necessary both for your comfort and to maintain an adequate milk supply. It can be accomplish most easily by using an electric breast pump, which can be rented from a surgical supply house. You can either save the milk to give to the baby at a later time or discard it. The baby can be fed stored breast milk or formula while you are at work and nursed as soon as you get home. Many mothers feel that this is a sure-fire mechanism to retain the closeness with their infant that they had before they returned to work.

Companies are slowly but surely recognizing that it is to their benefit to encourage breast-feeding. Indeed, according to the health insurer Kaiser Permanente, a formula-fed infant generates on average $1,435 more in medical expenses in his first six months than a breast-fed one. Sixteen percent of companies surveyed by the Society for Human Resource Management have some kind of lactation program, up from only 6 percent in 1999.

## Additional Resources

*Taking Care of Mom: A Guide to Postpartum* (Video)
Distributor: Injoy Productions
800-326-2082

*Mothering the Mother* (Book) by Marshall H. Claus, John H. Kennell, and Phyllis H. Klaus. Perseus Press, 1993

*Managing Career and Family*
Boxtree Communications
212-496-5600

National Partnership for Women and Families
1875 Connecticut Ave., NW
Washington, DC 20009
202-986-2600

Smart Moms, Healthy Babies
*www.smartmoms.org*

Pregnancy, Childbirth and Bladder Control
*www.niddk.nih.gov*

Doulas of North America (DONA)
13513 North Grove Drive
Alpine, UT 84004
801-756-7331
*www.dona.org*

# III

# Breast-feeding

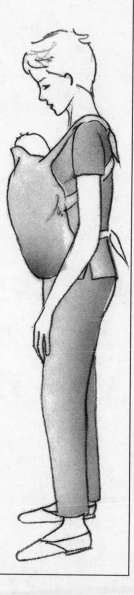

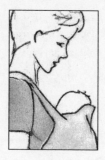

# 13

# Common Myths
# About Breast-feeding

In 1900, a newborn given something other than mother's milk had only one chance in ten of survival. Women breast-fed or paid for wet nurses. During World War I working-class women (the ones who often supplemented income through wet-nursing) went off to factory jobs, causing a shortage in wet nurses. Wealthy mothers had no choice but to breast-feed their babies themselves. But by 1950, technological progress in the agriculture and food industries permitted the development of cow's milk formula and only one baby in three was still fed at the breast.

Nearly all women have breasts "in working order." But breast-feeding is not instinctive—a few techniques must be learned. In the past, their mothers and grandmothers, who had the time and patience to accompany them through hours of nursing, taught new mothers. Today, this responsibility falls to a member of a hospital staff or a lactation consultant, who may be pressed for time.

The subject of breast-feeding is loaded with emotional connotations, because nursing has become a symbol of maternal love. Medical discoveries, new approaches, and even fashion trends have made it a widespread topic of discussion, and everyone has his or her two cents' worth to add to the debate. The result is that new mothers often feel incompetent and guilty if they encounter difficulties in breast-feeding. Therefore, we will try to set forth the issues as clearly as possible, so that your breast-feeding experience will run as smoothly and as satisfactorily as possible.

## The Importance of a Good Start

Successful nursing is in large part determined during the first week of the new infant's life. However, getting started is not always easy. Your milk may not come in on "schedule," some three days after delivery. It can come in as late as fifteen days after giving birth. The breasts can become engorged and painful. The baby may refuse to nurse for the first few days, or may fall asleep without having fed enough, then wake up shortly afterwards and require more. During the first few weeks, a new mother has not yet learned to "read" her baby's cries or know his rhythm and needs.

New mothers worry easily. Knowing that her infant is totally dependent on her, a mother naturally thinks: "I'm not feeding him correctly, I am a bad mother." During the first few weeks, stress-released hormones can also affect the milk supply, while later the mammary glands will function independently. Anxiety and the fear of failure can set off an inhibition mechanism, suppressing the milk supply: the mother then becomes even more frustrated, the baby becomes hungrier, and a vicious cycle begins. One negative remark is all it takes to discourage the mother. Then the bottle may seem to be the only solution.

All it takes, however, is patience, a bit of time, calm, and above all support from your friends and family, to overcome these early difficulties. Even though it is natural and instinctive, breast-feeding needs practice. Persevere, and give it time. The pleasure, well-being, and relaxation that nursing brings once it is fully underway is more than worth the trouble.

# The Truth Behind the Myths

In recent decades, American women have experienced great success with breast-feeding. But for the reluctant mother, or the new mother experiencing great difficulties, there can be tremendous peer pressure to continue what may seem to be an impossible task. In most cases, all that is needed is a strong support network and the confidence to proceed. Reassurance can be found in what follows.

### "Nursing Is Tiring"

Nursing is part of the body's natural postnatal process, allowing a gentler, more gradual hormonal change. Preventing lactation brutally breaks a normal evolutionary cycle. It is giving birth that is exhausting, and the whole postnatal period is also tiring. True, in the beginning, nursing requires you to be "on call" twenty-four hours a day, but choosing to become a mother means choosing to become available. Moreover, for the first month, a new mother really wants to be with her baby. Once nursing is well established (around four to six weeks), many women find it easier and more convenient than giving a bottle. They like the little pauses that nursing provides during the day. The endorphins that are released into a mother's body by nursing make her feel relaxed. And the satisfaction of seeing her baby grow and blossom thanks to her milk gives her great self-confidence. The ritual of stopping, sitting down, and taking time for her baby is pleasant and calming.

### "Nursing Ruins Your Breasts"

Pregnancy changes the breasts, as well as the rest of the body. "Maternity transforms one body into another." Inevitably, the skin will stretch and, in some cases, stretch marks may appear. But if women lose something purely aesthetic in becoming mothers, they gain greatly in physical maturity. In any case, it is the huge variations in weight and size (rapid weight gain, severe diets, engorgement, and certain hormonal treatments) that damage the breasts. Suddenly blocking milk production that has already begun is the worst thing you can do to the shape of your breasts. Nursing (especially for five or six months) provides a gentle return to normal, and helps to shape the contours of the breast.

### *"Formula Is Just as Good for Babies as Mother's Milk"*

This is false. A calf doubles his birth weight in ten weeks, whereas a baby takes twenty-four weeks to double his. The calf's body is completely formed at six months, the human being at sixteen years. Cow's milk must be very rich in protein and fat to satisfy the intense needs of the baby calf. A human baby can only use 86 percent of the elements contained in cow's milk, but can absorb 96 percent of the elements in his mother's milk. As a result, the baby digests mother's milk more easily: in forty-five to ninety minutes, as opposed to two or three hours for cow's milk. Maternal milk gives him enzymes to ease his digestion and metabolism. Because his liver, intestines, and kidneys are still immature, he needs the "ready-to-use" nutrients of breast milk. Mother's milk also contains certain fatty acids essential to the development of the brain during the first months of life.

Formula, even hypoallergenic milk that has been treated chemically to reduce potential allergic reactions, contains proteins that the newborn's intestines cannot digest. If these proteins enter the bloodstream, the baby's immune system will not recognize them and an allergic reaction can occur. It takes a hundred days for a baby's intestines, whose lining is very fine and fragile, to erect an efficient barrier against germs. This is doubtless the reason for the rise in milk allergies in children during the past twenty years. All it takes is one bottle to alter the intestinal flora and provoke an allergic reaction.

On the other hand, maternal milk contains IgA (Immunoglobulin A), antibodies that reinforce the baby's intestinal lining and make it impermeable to germs. For this reason, infants who are breast-fed have fewer gastric problems. In fact, the digestive process of human milk creates a chemical mixture which in turn creates an acidic environment in the digestive tract and kills bacteria. There is no bad maternal milk. If the baby is not getting fat, it is because he is not getting enough milk. It is important to remember that a breast-fed baby's growth curve may be less spectacular than a formula-fed baby may, because maternal milk does not cause as much water retention, nor the formation of fat cells as does formula.

### *"Failure at Breast-feeding May Unsettle an Emotionally Sensitive Woman"*

According to this logic, stopping nursing should restore a new mother's self-confidence and minimize her depression. But her emotional fragility and depression have many sources: hormonal, physical, socioeconomic, and psychological (see Chapters 17 and 18). Today, researchers are trying to develop antidepressants that allow depressed women to continue breast-feeding, because nursing is often one of their only sources of satisfaction.

### *"The Ability to Nurse Is Hereditary"* *(My Mother Couldn't So I Can't)*

This is absolutely untrue. But, if a woman has heard stories of failure all her life, she is likely to be less than confident at the beginning. Because milk production and milk flow are affected by stress during the early weeks, a nervous mother is advised to discuss her fears with specialists before giving birth. Midwives with lactation training and dedicated lactation organizations are available (many often work in conjunction with hospital staff). The new mother could also arrange for a specialist to be with her (even if only by telephone) during the first few weeks. Above all, she can talk to her baby, who already understands the intonations in his mother's voice.

### *"My Milk Is Not Rich Enough"*

Just as breast size has nothing to do with milk production, the color of milk has nothing to do with its nutritional value. For the first two weeks, the milk will be white as we imagine it should be, rich in sugars and fats. After the second or third week, it becomes more transparent, and even a little bluish. This is completely normal! Mother's milk is the food that is physiologically perfect for the newborn, perfectly adapted to his needs. It also changes throughout the day: it is more abundant and rich in fats in the morning. And it even changes during a single feeding session: milk contains four times as much fat at the end of a feeding than it does at the beginning. If the baby does not seem satisfied, it is because he is not eating enough. Do not forget that it takes about six weeks before the baby can strike a balance between his milk consumption and his real needs.

### *"It's Not Worth Starting to Breast-feed If I'm Returning to Work in a Few Weeks"*

Nursing a newborn infant during the first weeks is very different from nursing a two-month-old baby. Once the feeding pattern is established, a mother can leave the baby, even for a couple days, or nurse only morning and evening, by pumping milk at the office. Her milk production will no longer be affected by her emotions, but it will, however, be affected by her fatigue.

### *"It Is Impossible to Get Thin Again as Long as I'm Nursing"*

Because it is highly inadvisable for a woman to diet while nursing, the new mother will probably not be able to get back into her old clothes for a few months. But nursing—if continued for at least three months— is the only time in your life when the body burns up the fat in the thighs; fat that is often impossible to dislodge with a diet. Also, studies show that women who nurse for ten weeks lose an average of two pounds more than women who stop nursing after ten days. One warning, however: nursing is not an excuse to eat sweets or fatty food. . . .

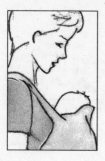

# 14

# Breast-feeding: Getting Off to a Good Start

## How the Breasts Produce Milk

For nine months, the volume of the breasts increases, as does that of the nipples and aureoles. The veins on the breasts become more apparent and a few drops of *colostrum* (a thick, yellow-tinted liquid) may form. During pregnancy, the interaction of several hormones prepares the breasts for nursing. *Estrogen* promotes growth in the mammary glands and also the proliferation of alveoli. *Progesterone* allows the mammary glands to mature. *Prolactin*, another lactation hormone, transforms cells in the breast into "secreting" cells, which will produce milk, and "muscular" cells, which will push the milk into the milk ducts (galactophoric channels).

During pregnancy, the twenty or so milk ducts in each breast will grow bunches at one end that are called *acini*. Each *acinus*, which resembles a raspberry, is nourished by a number of small, thin blood vessels (capillaries). Under the influence of the hormone prolactin, the blood flow to the breasts increases. Under this additional pressure, all the necessary ingredients for milk production are transferred from the blood vessels to the miniature milk production "factories" housed in the

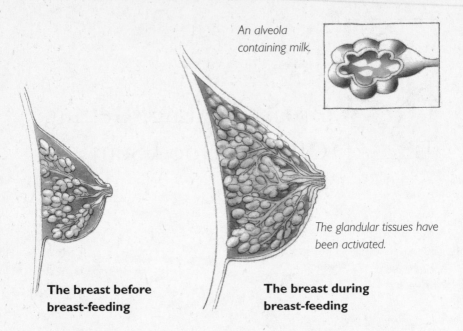

An alveola
containing milk.

The glandular tissues have
been activated.

**The breast before
breast-feeding**

**The breast during
breast-feeding**

acini. Thus the whole system is already in place during pregnancy, but kept on hold by the inhibiting influence of progesterone. Only a small amount of "birth milk," called colostrum, is allowed to accumulate.

With the expulsion of the placenta, the new mother's estrogen and progesterone levels drop. Prolactin takes over, and begins to stimulate milk production. A second hormone, *oxytocin*, commands the thousands of tiny muscle fibers enveloping the acini to squeeze them like oranges so as to push drops of milk into the milk ducts. The canals, in turn, also contract to eject the milk. Women are often surprised to find that milk comes out of several holes, like a showerhead, rather than from the tip of their breast. This is the ejection reflex. As soon as an acinus is emptied, it gets to work producing new milk.

In addition to hormone action, a woman needs a second stimulus to produce milk: suction from the baby's mouth on the nipple. The suckling sensation sends a message to the mother's brain, and the brain blocks the flow of the hormone that normally inhibits milk production. Likewise, when the breasts are full, another signal orders the brain to stop secreting the inhibiting hormone, and thus to slow milk production. Thus milk is produced primarily during the nursing session.

The breasts are not reservoirs: if they are not stimulated by suction for two or three weeks, prolactin production stops, and so does milk production. By contrast, a woman nursing twins will produce twice as much prolactin. If the baby is a big eater and frequently empties his mother's breasts, a signal will tell the brain to produce less of the inhibiting hormone and increase milk production.

A woman's breasts adapt to her baby's needs, which are generally greatest at around three months.

## The First Week

The first week often determines the success of your breast-feeding experience. As soon as the delivery is accomplished, the breasts begin to secrete colostrum. Within twenty-four hours, they will become extremely sensitive. Between the second and fourth day after delivery (sometimes longer after a cesarean), milk production begins. In the beginning, the breasts tingle: some women describe the sensation like "wanting to scratch on the inside." The next sensation is one of diffused heat, which grows progressively stronger. Finally, the breasts swell and can double in size. The veins are clearly visible.

It is well worth your time to inform yourself about breast-feeding before giving birth. This way you can form your own opinion about the task ahead. Above all, talk to your partner about your desire to breast-feed. You need his support. Some men do not take well to seeing their wife nursing.

So as to line up everything possible on your side, you need:

+ A good guidebook on breast-feeding.
+ The name of one or two friends who have successfully nursed their babies.
+ The phone number of a lactation consultant associated with your hospital or a breast-feeding support organization (see page 193).

## The Golden Rules

### Putting the Baby on the Breast Early

Even recently, newborns were separated from their mothers for twenty-four to forty-eight hours, during which time they received only a bit of sugar water. Fortunately, more and more doctors and midwives realize the importance of *colostrum* (the substance secreted by the breasts before the milk comes in) during the baby's first hours. Colostrum has a laxative effect and also helps prevent jaundice in the newborn. Furthermore, putting the baby to the breast early helps the mother also, because the baby's suction stimulates the production of oxytocin, the hormone that causes uterine contractions. The uterus gets back into shape much more quickly, and the risk of hemorrhaging decreases considerably.

It is during the first two hours of life that most babies suckle best. A few minutes after birth, babies already know how to crawl up their mother's belly, find a nipple, and suckle correctly. But this reflex disappears in six hours! Shortly thereafter, the baby enters a phase of "R&R," a type of sleepiness that lasts two days and makes the first nursing session much more difficult. Some babies are just not in a rush to nurse because they are tired from the birth process and drowsy from the medication that may have been given to their mother. They may wake up half an hour after birth and accept the breast, or it may be forty-eight hours later. The important thing is to let the baby choose his moment, and not to force him to take the nipple.

Immediately after birth, a baby needs colostrum. Because of its "laxative" effect, colostrum helps the baby discharge *meconium*, the

## MAKING SURE THAT YOUR NEEDS ARE HEARD

Tell the midwife or doctor that you want the baby given to you as soon as he is born, and put on your belly (the most reassuring spot for him, because he will hear the familiar sounds of your body), so you can nurse right on the delivery table, unless the baby needs urgent medical attention.

If the staff changes shift while you are still in the labor room, do not hesitate to tell the new nurses your wishes.

Ask your partner to help make sure that your requests are carried out. Even if before you give birth he thinks these requests seem unimportant, he will probably be so shaken up by the delivery that he will do everything he can to make sure your needs are met. He should also be warned, however, that if there is an emergency the baby may have to be taken away quickly and you will not be allowed to nurse.

dead cell matter that accumulated in his intestines while in utero. Colostrum also gives the baby energy reserves, because it contains sugars that he can use immediately. In addition, it provides proteins and mineral salts that will help the baby retain the water necessary for his own hydration. He will lose less weight during the days following his birth. Finally, colostrum carries important antibodies that will provide the baby with precious protection against infection.

## Feeding on Demand

For at least six weeks, a newborn does not differentiate between day and night, hunger and sleepiness. You therefore cannot impose daytime and nighttime schedules on him. He can sleep without being fed, and may cry even if he has had enough to eat. Little by little, his mother will learn to tell the difference between his calls for food and his other cries (fatigue, overstimulation, cold, pain, etc.). We have all heard of the baby who sleeps through the night from the day that he leaves the hospital. Unfortunately, this is the exception.

**Feeding on demand does not mean you are becoming a slave to your baby. It means you are helping him develop a rhythm of eating and sleeping.**

Deciding to give your child the incomparable advantage of maternal milk does mean making a commitment to establishing your nursing routine. That means accepting that nursing comes before any other task, that for a few weeks your clock may be completely different from that of those around you. It is therefore vital to have organized your family's daily life, and any household needs, before the baby's birth.

Newborns feed at least eight times a day. Their feeding sessions last from 20 to 45 minutes. Mother's milk can be digested in twenty minutes or in two hours. The number of feedings can vary from one day to the next, and from one child to another. So in the beginning you need to be available, day and night. You will not have more milk by making a hungry baby wait. On the contrary, if you let the infant choose his own feeding schedule and dictate the length of each session, you are assured of always having enough milk. At three months, a baby who was fed on demand sleeps just as well and just as long as a baby that was subjected to severe discipline.

## A FEW TIPS

Do not wake the baby to feed (except during the first week to prevent engorgement, or if the baby is premature, or if he sleeps more than five hours).

Give him your breast only when he asks for it.

Let him feed as long as he wants to (see below for how to differentiate feeding and sucking for pleasure or pacifying).

## Your Position

This is probably the most important factor for preventing pain and soreness, and therefore for getting off to a good start. A new mother spends at least three hours a day—and sometimes much more—breast-feeding. If she is sitting uncomfortably, she will get cramps and may injure her back. In addition, painful cracks may appear on the nipples if the baby is badly positioned: the breast is pulled in the wrong direction, and the tension is badly distributed.

## Getting Comfortable

The "classic" position that we see in artworks or in advertisements (the mother seated, with the baby tucked in at her elbow) is difficult to imitate if you are sitting up in bed and even harder to do if you have had a cesarean or have a painful episiotomy scar. The newborn does not have good muscle coordination and needs to be guided, which is difficult to do if he is hidden in your elbow. Here are some more efficient positions, especially for the first days.

**Lying down**: This is the best position for nursing in bed at night (when you can snooze or even sleep while the baby is feeding!), after a cesarean, or if you have a painful episiotomy scar. Lie down on your side, with the baby against your belly, propping both of you up on pillows. Lift your breast a bit so the baby can latch on correctly.

**Seated:** As soon as you can, it is preferable to nurse in an armchair (seated on your special cushion or a child's buoy if you are uncomfortable), propped up by as many cushions as it takes to keep your back straight. Put your feet on a footstool or a pile of books, and place a pillow on your lap so that the baby is as high as your breasts. Avoid leaning forward.

You can hold the baby with the arm opposite to the breast he is feeding on, placing him on a cushion or two on your lap. This way, your arm supports his back, while your hand supports the back of his head and his neck. His face is directly in front of the breast.

You can also hold the baby on the side, like a chick under the hen's wing. This position is recommended after a cesarean, or with twins. Place cushions against the arms of the chair and "seat" the baby so that he faces the chair's back. Bring his face to the front of your breast while supporting his back with your arm and his head with the palm of your hand, your thumb behind one of his ears and your index finger behind his other ear.

The baby's tummy should be against your body, his chin against his own chest, and his mouth must be exactly placed at the tip of your breast. You must feel completely at ease: the baby's weight should not rest on your arm or cause tension in your back or shoulders. Use cushions to raise the baby to the right height. Above all, he should not pull on your breast.

Before starting to nurse, make some large circles with your shoulders, from front to back, so as to rid yourself of tension. Inhale when your shoulders are back, and exhale when they are forward. Keep breathing while your are nursing. Often, women have trouble getting the milk going because they don't breathe deeply enough.

## The Feed

### Latching on

Compress the breast with the thumb and index finger (at the "8 o'clock" and "2 o'clock" positions on your breast) behind the *areola*. Gently brush the baby's mouth with the nipple until he opens up his mouth wide. Do not forget that it is mainly the odor of the small sebaceous glands surrounding the nipple (*Montgomery ducts*) which catch the newborn's attention. Gently bring his head toward the breast when his mouth is wide open. Be sure that the areola is fully inside his mouth, and that his lower lip is out. When he starts to feed, let go of your breast. It is not necessary to keep your finger on your breast to "unblock" the baby's nose. His nostrils are under the protuberance of his nose, and he will be able to breathe normally. However, if you cre-

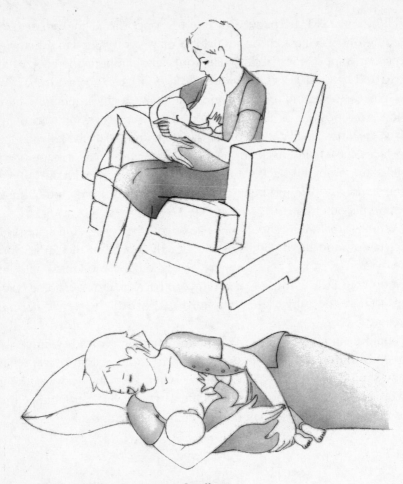

**The correct position for breast-feeding**
*Whether sitting or lying down, the baby's stomach should be parallel to yours, with his head positioned at the same angle as your breast*

ate tension pushing against your breast, you will be pulling the fragile tissues and may cause cracks to develop. If the breast is really too soft or too large, place your hand in a wreath shape under the breast to give it a convex shape.

Unlike adults, babies know how to swallow with their tongue far forward: the tongue plays the role of a conduit to guide the milk spray towards his throat. You should not hear clicking sounds (which would mean he is playing with his tongue) and the baby's cheeks should not suck inwards. If the baby seems to be positioned badly, don't hesitate to place his mouth back on in a better position. If he is in the wrong position, he will not be able to swallow easily. Not wanting to suffocate, he will pull on the breast to "reposition" the nipple. This strong, asymmetric position will tear fragile tissues in the tip of the breast, and will cause cracking of the nipples.

When you want the baby to switch sides, it is nearly impossible (and very painful) to pull the nipple out of his mouth. A baby's suction is incredibly powerful. Push down on his chin to make him open his mouth, or slide a (clean!) finger into the corner of his mouth. You will hear, and feel, the suction being released.

## The Letdown Reflex

It is the baby who "makes" his milk. He needs to suck for a few moments (sometimes a few minutes, during the first days, or if the surrounding atmosphere is agitated) before the signal to "open the dams" reaches your brain. This is the ejection or "letdown" reflex: the milk then will begin to spurt out. Then, the baby consumes 50 percent of his rations in the first two minutes, and 80 to 90 percent in the first four minutes of nursing.

At the beginning of the feeding, the milk is composed mainly of water and mineral salt, which will quench the baby's thirst, as well as carbohydrates, which promote the growth of *lactobacillus*, whose role is to consolidate the antiinfectious barrier in his intestine. By the middle of the feeding session, the milk contains more proteins and fats. It is near the end of the session when the milk becomes "richer": now it contains larger fat globules and proteins, which take longer to come down the milk ducts. This last form of milk makes the baby feel sated and signals to him that the meal is over. The last 20 percent of the baby's ration, which comes after the first five minutes, is therefore very important. Moreover, the baby needs to suckle, and the feeding session gives him so much pleasure that he may stay on the breast for 20 or 30 minutes. It is this pleasure deriv d from suckling, as much as the caloric contents, that satisfies the baby.

In the case of twins, it is better to feed them together, or to separate their feeding times by an hour, because the milk flow lasts for only 20 minutes.

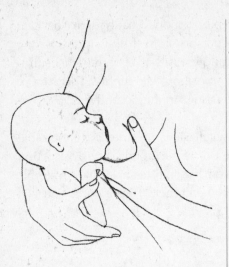
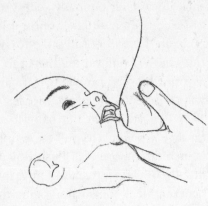

**YES**                            **NO**

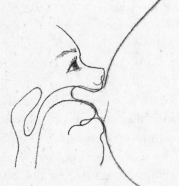
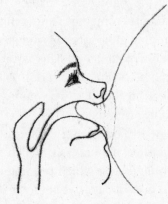

The baby grabs the entire areola, not just the nipple. The nipple will be drawn all the way to the middle of his palate. His tongue will continually flick back and forth to stimulate the sensory receptors of the areola while forming a conduit for the milk to flow in to his throat.

The baby is only sucking the nipple, which does not extend far enough into his mouth. The sensory receptors are not sufficiently stimulated. Therefore the signal to begin the production of milk is not strong enough.

## How Do You Know When the Baby Has Finished Feeding?

Listen to the "gulps" he makes while swallowing the milk. During the first series of gulps, while he is getting his principal nourishment, there will be twenty or so "gulps," followed by a pause of two or three minutes (even though he may still be sucking). A second flux begins, although slightly less long and less powerful, followed by another, longer pause. This rhythm of fluxes and pauses continues. At the end of the fourth flux, there is almost no more milk. Nevertheless, do not underestimate the pleasure that the baby is getting while suckling, even if the nourishing part of the feeding is over. During the first days, the baby must determine for himself the ratio of milk, sleep, and pleasure that suits him best. If you are not pressed for time, let him suckle just for fun. Contrary to what some misinformed people may tell you, sore nipples are not due to long feeding sessions, they are due to bad positioning.

During the first days, before the breasts have become accustomed to the baby's powerful sucking, new mothers are strongly advised to nurse frequently. (The prolactin necessary for milk production only needs forty-five minutes to an hour to reconstitute itself.) Nurse for short periods only, and change sides so that the baby suckles on both breasts. Remember which side you started on, so that at the next feed, you can start on the other side. Because newborns tire quickly, it is good to make them switch breasts five to ten minutes after the ejection reflex. Later, it is preferable to wait for the baby to let go by himself before offering him the second breast.

In the past, some hospitals advised mothers to pump the rest of their milk after a feeding, or to manually stimulate their breasts so as to "empty them completely." Now, we recognize that this is not only useless, it is aggressive, and damages the breast's delicate tissues. Breasts are not reservoirs, so they do not need to be "emptied." It is only by putting the baby to your breast regularly and often during the first days that you can prevent engorgement and ensure that your milk will come in abundantly.

**Alternating sides is good stimulation for the breasts. And it can often wake up a drowsy baby.**

Try to nurse in calm surroundings. In the brain, the limbic system, the command and control center for our emotions, is located next to the hypothalamus, the body's clock that regulates all our rhythms: sleeping/waking, hormonal secretions, cardiac and respiratory rhythms, hunger, weight, and the menstrual period. If you are upset, tense, or angry, the limbic system will block production of the oxytocin necessary to eject milk. This reflex dates from a prehistoric era, when a mother had to be able to flee from a saber-toothed tiger without being burdened by milk running from her breasts. Fortunately, a mother's body "forms habits," and the milk production reflex becomes far less dependent on emotions by the end of a few weeks.

But during the crucial starting up phase, it is particularly important to nurse in a calm atmosphere. Often, visitors bring neither the relaxation nor the emotional support that a new mother needs. We advise you to choose one or two people who are close to you who have successfully breast-fed and whom you trust, and only listen to them. Smile politely to the others, but don't respond. They usually tire of giving advice and making comments after a short while.

+ After each feeding session, take time to get the tension knots out of your neck and shoulders: stretch your arms above your head, make circles with your shoulders, and rotate your neck, massage your upper back, look at the ceiling, try to stretch your spine, take long, deep breaths.
+ Drink your fill. Limiting your fluid intake will not prevent engorgement. Drinking a huge amount does not make more milk. A nursing mother is naturally more thirsty.
+ Eat at night. Milk production is a twenty-four-hour-a-day business. So you must nourish yourself day and night. Lowfat yogurt and dried fruits are particularly good midnight snacks.
+ Wear a nursing bra day and night.
+ Keep the baby near you, or make sure that the nurses will bring him to you when he cries. Do not hesitate to take him into your bed, even in the hospital.

It is normal to feel uterine contractions while you nurse, throughout the first week (see pages 28 to 29 for tips on easing the pain). The contractions are brought on by the body producing oxytocin to eject the milk. You may also notice more blood on your sanitary pad after a feeding session.

Breasts often "overflow" in the beginning, because oxytocin production is not yet well regulated. One breast can overflow while the baby is nursing at the other one. The breasts can also start flowing if the mother hears her baby crying. Heat, altitude, or emotions also affect the reflex. Some women use breast-feeding cups to gather this milk and save it. It is also helpful to wear nursing pads inside your bra to avoid leaks.

Try not to pump your milk in the beginning, unless your baby cannot nurse for medical reasons. Pumping risks provoking an overproduction of milk. But once the baby's feeding pattern is established, the breast pump is a valuable ally, which will allow you to be more independent while still providing your baby (and you) the benefits of mother's milk. Try to pump in the morning, when supply is greatest (right after the day's first feed).

Sometimes, the milk can flow too quickly, and the baby chokes or appears to have difficulty swallowing. He gets discouraged, refuses the breast, and then cries because he is hungry half an hour later. In this case, it is important to hold him as vertically as possible (unfortunately, the lying-down position is not advised) and to calm him, to encourage him to suckle less avidly. Above all, do not abandon him! The baby will learn to pull less energetically to regulate the milk flow.

Avoid letting your nipples dry out. Do not wash your breasts with soap in the shower or bath, just rinse with water. Do not wash them before and after every feeding session (as is still advised in some hospitals), and do not dry them with a hair dryer. Simply leave them exposed and let them air-dry. Maternal milk is an excellent disinfectant, and also has the advantages of being edible and healing to the skin. It is useless to clean it off. You can, however, rub pure lanolin (but not a lanolin-based cream) on the nipples. You can also use a vitamin A- or E-based ointment.

It is normal for the breasts to be suppler in the evening. It does not mean that you have less milk.

Sometimes, the baby prefers one breast to the other. There are many reasons for this: he can hear your heart beating on the left side; if you are right-handed, you hold him better on that side; you put a bit too much cream on one nipple; your shirt bothers him . . . to get him to accept the "wrong" side, keep him in the same position while you slip him from one breast to the other, or put him in front of it sitting up and talk to him about the fact that you wish that he would nurse at that breast.

Before you leave the hospital be sure that you have asked the

---

### IMPROVING YOUR MILK PRODUCTION

**Homeopathy**

Ricinus 4C is recommended. Take 4 granules morning and evening between thirty-six and seventy-two hours after giving birth. Beware however that though this remedy is effective, it may also cause nausea and diarrhea. If this occurs, replace it with 3 granules Sabal Serrulata 4C three times a day.

**Herbal Remedies**

The following herbs support lactation: Comfrey, Milk Thistle, Red Clover, Alfafa, Nettles, Fenugreek, and Hops. Drink 4 or 5 cups of infusion of a combination of these herbs per day (30 to 40 grams of herbs/dried flowers per quart of water).

**Aromatherapy**

3 drops essential oil of Fennel on a sugar cube or a spoonful of honey. This is equivalent to drinking 1 gallon fennel tea.

---

nurses and lactation consultants all the questions that come to your mind. Once home, do not hesitate to call the hospital "warm line" or lactation staff if you have any further need of assistance.

## Breast-feeding Problems

### Supplements and Formula

Mixing formula from a bottle and nursing in the first few weeks is the surest way to cause breast-feeding to fail. The way a baby sucks on a bottle is completely different from the way he suckles a breast. The baby must pinch the sides of a silicone or rubber nipple to make the milk flow. He has to swallow like an adult, keeping his tongue inside his mouth. Some babies suffer from "nipple confusion" and have a very hard time distinguishing an artificial nipple from a real one. They choke, get angry, and often end up refusing the breast, which requires more of an effort than the bottle from which the milk flows by itself. (This confusion will generally end after three or four weeks.)

Formula holds a newborn longer (up to four hours instead of three) because it is less easily digested than mother's milk. If the baby receives a supplement, he will be less hungry at the next feeding time. He will therefore take less milk and become hungry again shortly thereafter. All your breast-feeding efforts will be undone, and you will run the risk of engorgement. The breasts, less stimulated, will produce less milk. The baby will be hungry. You will be tempted to give him another bottle. And your lactation will start to fade.

You must insist, gently but firmly, that no one give your baby a bottle. In the hospital, if supplementing with formula is still practiced, you will have to remind the new nurse on every shift, because her predecessor will probably not have passed on the message. You can stick a little sign on the baby's isolette that says something like: "Hello! If I am crying, take me to my mommy. I don't drink formula." You can also choose to keep the baby in your room instead of in the nursery, ask to have "rooming in."

## THE BABY IS FEEDING ENOUGH

*If*

- Your milk has come in by the third or fourth day after childbirth.
- The baby nurses at least eight times in a twenty-four-hour period (about every two or three hours, except for a fairly common five-hour sleeping session in the night).
- The baby nurses for between ten and fifteen minutes each time, and seems satisfied, even if he has not fallen asleep.
- He swallows ("gulps") every three or four sucks. If he only swallows three or four times per minute, he might not be getting enough milk. You must then stimulate your production by getting him to nurse more often.
- He falls asleep calmly, completely relaxed, with his fingers spread apart.
- Your breasts feel lighter and damp after a nursing session.
- The baby wets between six and eight diapers per day (he will urinate more often from the fifth day on) and has at least three bowel movements per day (but six or eight stools per day is also normal, and is not a sign of diarrhea). Starting from the fifth day, or even earlier, his movements are golden yellow, fairly liquid and grainy, with a sweet odor. Later, when the nursing is really underway, some babies digest maternal milk so well that they only have a bowel movement every second day!

During the early weeks, when the mother has not yet learned to recognize her baby's different cries, she can confuse the traditional nighttime crying with cries of hunger. Her first reaction is to assume that she does not have enough milk, and to offer him a bottle.

## Sleepy Babies

Most newborns, as we have seen, are in a recuperation phase for the first days after their birth. Premature babies and babies with jaundice can remain very sleepy even longer. This state can make breast-feeding difficult and frustrating. Make sure the baby can smell your nipples—avoid cleaning them with alcohol or any other disinfectant. Put a few drops of colostrum or milk on his lips, rub his back, tug gently on his earlobes, tickle his feet, and talk to him. Sometimes, a cool (but not cold) washcloth will rouse him. Insist that the nursing staff bring the baby to you every three hours and do not give him a bottle—even if it is of your milk—until you have tried for 24 hours without success.

## Difficulty in Latching On

Nursing is a technique that the baby must also master. Some babies are born with a sucking mechanism not yet fully developed. Others choke a bit and cannot swallow the milk as quickly as they are drawing it. These problems will disappear with time. You just have to have courage to persevere and to ask for help and advice, first in the hospital and then from lactation organizations when you get back home.

## Engorgement

Engorgement is a swelling of the breasts caused by the congestion of blood flow into the area combined with insufficient drainage. This is a relatively common problem that occurs during the first few days after your milk comes in, when the production is not yet stabilized. The arrival of milk on the second or third day after giving birth provokes a dramatic dilation of the breast's vascular network. Only the lactation mechanism (making and then ejecting milk) can reduce the tension in the veins. If the breasts are regularly and properly stimulated (eight to ten times a day), and if the mother feels comfortable, the risks of engorgement are negligible. But if the breasts are not sufficiently

## A FEW TIPS

It is not uncommon for babies to suddenly refuse one breast or both some time during the first week. First, check to make sure that no one gave him a bottle. And here are a few "tips" to remedy the situation.

- If your breasts seem hard and engorged, soften the areola just before nursing by drawing a little milk manually (under a hot shower, if necessary).
- If the baby moves his head from side to side, hold it against your breast so his tongue can feel the nipple.
- Have him suck your finger for a few seconds before bringing him to your breast.
- If the baby seems to "spit back" the breast, put an ice cube on your nipple for a few minutes to firm it up.
- If the baby seems to be swallowing his tongue rather than sucking the nipple, check to see whether his frenulum (the small membrane under the tongue) is not too short. A doctor can remedy this.
- Try every half-hour. After several fruitless attempts, pump your milk to maintain your production. Try to resist giving him your milk in a bottle for at least twenty-four hours. Some babies take ten days to learn how to nurse.

A 1991 study showed that garlic in the mother's diet dramatically improved babies suckling time! Not only does garlic have an antiseptic effect, but also babies sucked more efficiently and for longer periods when their milk was "flavored" with garlic.

drained, they will become tender and warm and the swelling and increased pressure will hinder the flow of milk. Inflammation may even cause fever or lumps to appear in the armpits.

If you are tempted to sleep throughout the night and have someone else feed your baby, do not forget that prolactin, the milk production hormone, is secreted most abundantly during the first part of the night, during your phases of deep sleep. Night feedings are therefore indispensable during the first days to prevent engorgement.

It can also happen that a new mother is successfully breast-feeding in the hospital, but when she gets home (especially if she left the hospital quickly) her rhythms are perturbed. Her breasts become hard and the baby has a hard time suckling. If this happens to you, by all means do not give up! Follow the advice given below, and give yourself forty-eight hours of complete rest.

### A Few Suggestions for Relieving Engorgement

+ Wear a supportive nursing bra at all times.
+ Shower in warm water (not too hot) and apply warm water compresses to the breasts, particularly before feedings.
+ Maintain frequent feeding sessions (almost every hour) which last at least ten minutes on each side. Gently rub the sore area of your breast after the feeding session.
+ Apply compresses of powdered aspirin or gently rub the breasts with an anti-inflammatory ointment (such as Ben-Gay, which athletes use on sore muscles). Cover the breasts with a thick piece of cotton wool and wrap them loosely with an Ace bandage for up to three hours at a time (during the baby's longest nap). Be sure to wash them well before nursing.
+ Manually express some milk before the feeding session to get the milk flowing and relieve pressure, as well as to help the baby grasp the areola more easily. Under a warm shower, place your fingers on the edges of the areola, the thumb above it, the other fingers below. Push hard directly toward your chest, then release while rolling your thumb and fingers toward the nipple, as though you were making fingerprints. Continue in a rhythmic manner: push, roll, push, and roll, to empty the breast enough so that the baby can easily take the nipple in his mouth. Avoid pulling on the nipple itself or compressing the breast.

## Pain

Sometimes, breast-feeding seems to go well in the beginning, and then suddenly, two or three days later, the nipples become very sensitive. The pain will usually disappear after about ten feedings or so, but it can last three or four days. For other women, nursing can be painful during the first few seconds of a feeding session, but the pain goes away quickly.

## How to Get Beyond These Difficult First Days?

+ Take acetaminophen (Tylenol) half an hour before breast-feeding. This poses no risk for the baby.
+ Massage the tip of your breast with an ice cube for a few minutes before nursing so as to numb it a bit. The pain diminishes, to a large extent, once the milk is flowing.
+ Remember that the "training period" can be uncomfortable but short-lived. For the baby's well-being, for the beauty of your own breasts (ceasing to nurse while the milk is coming in can damage the shape of your breasts), and to avoid any possibility of infection, this is not the moment to give up! If you can hang on for a few weeks, breast-feeding will become a pleasure and you will feel no pain at all.

## Chapping

For the first two or three weeks of breast-feeding, the nipples can become chapped (when the nipple is marked with tiny red traces) or crack. The tip or the base can look bright red or raspberry red. The pain is intense, and it will bleed (small amounts) often. But the most serious disadvantage is that the wounds can become an entryway for germs. Bad positioning of the baby, who pinches or pulls on the nipple, causes cracked nipples. They can also be caused by dampness or overdrying of the skin.

To prevent cracking, check that your nursing position is perfect. From the very first sessions, ask the nurse to stay with you to watch how the baby latches on. For the first forty-eight hours, a baby nurse or a maternity nurse with lactation training should be at your side to verify that the baby is taking the nipple correctly. Wash your hands before each feed. Let your breasts dry in the open air—try not to cover them with a bra or a shirt—for half an hour after the feeding session.

In case of a cracked nipple, wipe some of your fresh milk on the wound. Your milk is one of the best antiseptics known to science. Change your nursing pad frequently, and avoid greasy ointments that promote dampness. Even though they are controversial, silicone nipple covers can be helpful. But try not to use them very long. You may, if necessary, rest your nipples for six to twelve hours, nursing the baby on one side only and drawing milk from the resting nipple with your

## A FEW TIPS

- Empty the breasts 10 to 12 times every 24 hours, starting with the unhealthy side. This will be painful in the beginning, but the pain will diminish once the breast has been emptied a bit.
- Between feedings, apply hot, moist compresses (you can add crushed aspirin to the compresses), covered in cotton wool. Another option recommended by herbalists is to apply very green cabbage leaves to your breasts, inside your nursing bra. Leave them in until they become wet. They will draw the heat out of your breasts.
- Observe strict bed rest, with the baby at your side.
- Some women feel that applying cold gives more comfort than heat. If you prefer, apply an ice pack, well wrapped in a towel so as not to burn your breast with the cold.

By following this advice, your symptoms should disappear in twenty-four to forty-eight hours. But if the problem persists for more than thirty-six hours, call your doctor, because you should start an antibiotic treatment that is compatible with breast-feeding. You will have to follow the course of antibiotics for ten to fifteen days. Do not stop taking them before the full course is finished, because a relapse can cause an abscess in the breast. If at all possible, you should continue breast-feeding to keep the milk flowing and avoid clogging. After each feeding the infected breast should be thoroughly emptied either by hand or with a pump, if the baby has not done a complete job himself.

hand (not with a breast pump!) every three hours to maintain production. If the crack is not too big, you can continue to nurse the baby by placing him at a 90-degree angle from his habitual position so as to change the pressure on your breast.

## Mastitis

Another common problem associated with breast-feeding is mastitis. This is an infection of the breast tissue that often affects first-time mothers during the early weeks of nursing. It is usually caused by germs that enter into a milk duct through a crack in the skin of the nipple. Early warning signs that precede infection include engorge-

---

### MASTITIS

**Herbal Remedies**

- Hot compresses of Parsley or Comfrey (tie a handful of leaves in an old piece of cotton and immerse in simmering water for ten minutes; then allow to cool until you can just tolerate the heat before applying to breasts).
- Immerse breasts in an infusion of Marshmallow Root and Fennel Seeds (prepared and left to stand overnight before reheating and left to cool)
- For stubborn cases, take 20 to 40 drops of Purple Cane Flower tincture at hourly intervals.

---

ment, elevated temperature, and localized tenderness in one breast. These symptoms should be treated promptly to avoid infection. Once actual infection has set in, it is marked by a sudden rise in temperature of 102 to 104°F, intense fatigue, shivers, overall body soreness, painful mammary swelling, and a red tender area on the breast. It is important to contact your doctor or midwife immediately for treatment.

### To Prevent Mastitis

+ Nurse frequently to avoid engorgement.
+ Avoid chapping by nursing in a good position, letting your nipples dry in open air, being sure not to irritate the nipples with aggressive products, and keeping your breasts dry.
+ Avoid drafts. Always cover your chest and arms.

*Warning:* repeated bouts of mastitis may often be due to the same infection which has never been completely cured. Sometimes it corresponds to a vitamin C deficiency, anemia, or even simply wearing a bra that is too tight.

## Breast Abscess

This is a very rare complication that develops when mastitis is left untreated. It appears as a high fever and lancing or throbbing pain in the breast that feels like a hard, painful lump. The mother is exhausted and very pale. Treatment includes a course of antibiotics and often a

## REMEDIES FOR PROBLEM NURSING

### Weak Milk Production

#### Homeopathy
- Take 3 granules Ricinus 4C three times a day in combination with:
  - Agnus Castus 5C if you feel tired and sad.
  - Asa Foetida 5C if your nipples are red and sensitive, and the veins on your breast are very noticeable.
- Drink 4 or 5 cups of Fennel tea per day. Make this with 30 to 40 grams of Fennel flowers per quart of water.

#### Aromatherapy
- Before lunch take 10 drops of a mixture that is equal parts essential oils of Wheat, Barley, and Oats on a lump of sugar or a spoonful of honey.

### Engorgement

#### Homeopathy
- Take 3 granules Phytolacca 7C three times a day for two days, then Phytolacca 9C for two days.
- Take Urtica Urens 5C if your breasts are engorged and painful.
- If you think you are producing too much milk, which provokes engorgement pain, 3 granule Lac Caninum 5C in the morning can bring relief.
- Pulsatilla 30C four times daily for one week can decrease engorgement. If you want to stop breast-feeding, it will slow then stop your milk supply in 200C strength. But at 5C strength it will help restore your milk supply after suppression due to an infection.
- For lumpy, hard breasts, Phytolacca is recommended in order to heal congestion before it becomes infected.

#### Herbal Remedies
- Cold compresses of essential oil of Peppermint are helpful, but remember to wipe your breasts carefully before nursing.

## Pain During Nursing

### Homeopathy

- If your nipples are sore and smarting: Arnica Montana 5C.
- If your nipples are very sensitive to the touch and you are very tense: Chamomilla 5C.
- If the nipples are red and sensitive: Croton Tiglium 5C.
- If the pain occurs only after the baby has started to nurse: Rhus Toxicodendron 5C, or Silica 5C if there is a sharp pain when the baby latches on.
- If the pain is located particularly on the right side of the breast, and then radiates to the other breast, or if you have too much milk and you are tense: Borax 5C.
- If, when the baby is nursing, the pain radiates through your body and you feel a lump under your armpit: Phytolacca 5C.
- If the pain seems to be coming from inside the breast and radiates toward your back: Phellandrium 5C.

## Cracked Nipples (Chapping)

### Homeopathy

- To fight cracked nipples, alternate the following remedies four times a day: 5 granules Nitricum Acidum 5C and Graphites 15C; then take any of the following remedies, depending on your condition:
  - If the cracks are accompanied by intense pain during nursing: Phytolacca 5C.
  - If the skin on the nipple is cracked and tends to ooze: Petroleum 5C, or Hepar Sulphuris 5C (especially if there is pus).
  - If the nipple is chapped and ulcerated: Castor Equisetum 4C.
  - If the cracks produce a runny yellow substance that looks like honey: Graphites 5C.
  - If the cracks are bleeding: Nitricum Acidum 5C.
  - If you feel a strong pain in the breast during feeding that radiates to your shoulder: Croton Tiglium 5C.
  - If in addition to cracked nipples you suffer from headaches and constipation: Lac Defloratum 5C.

Homeopaths also recommend lightly massaging the nipples with Castor Equi Cream.

continued on next page

### Herbal Remedies
- Compresses dipped in an infusion of Marigold or Comfrey provide relief. Ointments made from Comfrey or Yarrow also are available in some health food stores. Aloe Vera gel is helpful but leaves a bitter taste for the baby.
- Herbalists recommend placing Geranium leaves (underside against your skin) inside your bra to soothe and heal cracked nipples.

## Mastitis

### Homeopathy
- Take 3 granules Silicea 30C twice a day until the symptoms disappear.
  - Or else 3 granules Phytolacca 7C three times a day for the first day, then 9C the second day, and finally 12C the third day.
- If you are taking a classical allopathic medication for mastitis, you can complement it with:
  - 3 granules Pyrogenium 5C taken once a day.
  - 3 granules Belladonna 4C twice a day.
  - 3 granules of Byronia Alba 9C every third day.
- If your breasts are very sensitive, congested, or bluish, and you have hot sweats: 3 granules Lachesis Multis 5C three times a day.
- If your fever is high and your condition is degrading: 3 granules Antracium 9C three times a day.
- If your pulse is rapid, if you are drained of energy, yet agitated at the same time: 3 granules Pyrogenium 9C three times a day.

## Breast Abscess

### Homeopathy
- As soon as the abscess begins to form, and the breast is red and hot, with throbbing pain: Belladonna Atropina 9C.
- If the abscess is oozing pus: Hepar sulphur 4C.
- If you have a tendency toward abscesses, take Silica 6C four times a day as a preventive measure. Silica is excellent for mastitis, abscesses, and internal infections as it promotes the extrusion of foreign bodies and healing.

surgical procedure to drain the abscess. You may continue to nurse on the healthy breast but must pump the affected breast until healing is complete and nursing can resume.

## Mother's Milk for Premature or Sick Babies

Premature or sick babies need their mother's milk even more than full-term babies do. Increasingly, neonatal units are encouraging mothers to breast-feed if at all possible. If your baby was born prematurely, keep in mind that he is not as strong as a full-term baby and therefore may suck with less ability. If you can nurse him directly, it is very important to position him so you can watch him suck (see page 164, "Lying down"). Premature babies tend to fall asleep quickly, and often need to be tickled gently to stay awake so that they get enough nourishment. They may not take much milk at each session but are frequently hungry (some mothers find that pumping out their breasts after the baby is finished nursing helps maintain their milk supply if they cannot be present in the neonatal unit for each feeding).

If you cannot breast-feed your baby directly, you can still provide him with your milk by using an electric breast pump. Your hospital may have some available for use by new mothers. Pumps can be bought or rented from pharmacies and many baby supply stores. It is worth investing in the purchase or rental of a high-quality pump in order to save time and avoid any unnecessary strain on your nipples (ideally, an electric pump that lets you pump both breasts at once). Even when pumping milk, it is helpful to maintain a schedule similar to that of the baby: at least eight times in a twenty-four-hour period, day and night. Unfortunately, you can't pump eight times during the day and sleep all night, because your milk production won't keep up with that schedule. In fact, the best pumping times are around midnight and the early hours of the morning, when the milk supply is highest. If you only pump during the day, your milk production inevitably will diminish. If your breast pump is mechanical, rather than electric, it is advisable to switch back and forth between breasts several times during the pumping session.

Pumped (or "expressed") milk will keep for forty-eight hours in the refrigerator or three months in the freezer. Often, a layer of yellowish "cream" will form on the surface. Just shake the milk before heating it to redistribute the "cream."

Here are a few tips for easy and efficient milk pumping:

+ Take a hot shower just before pumping.
+ Apply a warm compress to the breast just before pumping.
+ Gently massage the breast, from the center of your chest outward to the nipple.
+ Have someone massage your back during the pumping session.
+ Look at a photograph of your baby while you are pumping your milk.

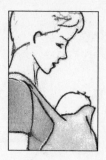

# 15

# An Established Routine

For the first two or three weeks, breast-feeding can seem fairly erratic: the baby does not yet differentiate night from day, and demands nourishment with no regular schedule. It is common for milk production to diminish when the new mother gets home from the hospital. But as soon as she returns to her old habits and can enjoy being back in her own house, production will resume fully.

Once she has returned home, the new mother will quickly come to realize that breast-feeding requires 100 percent availability for a few weeks. Ideally, she should have organized the running of her household well in advance of her delivery (see pages 100 to 104).

Fortunately, nursing gets easier and easier. Most mothers who nurse for more than three months will tell you that breast-feeding is more practical than carrying bottles and formula around. You should also know that, according to the World Health Organization (WHO), a baby needs no nourishment other than breast milk for the first six months of life. Unfortunately, we are often influenced by other people's ideas such as "you have to stop nursing before you go back to work" and are subjected to pressure from baby food companies.

# Integrating Breast-feeding into Your Routine

The two worst enemies of breast-feeding are fatigue and loneliness. If you begin to feel discouraged, do not hesitate to contact a lactation support organization (see page 193) and ask one of their representatives to pay you a house call.

Unfortunately, some women stop breast-feeding too early because they are afraid to nurse in public. Outside the house, they get dirty looks from people, as though they were no more than a cow. They then feel trapped at home, and excluded from any social life. But just think, standing up to other people's disapproval when you are breast-feeding is just the beginning. Later, people will comment on how you dress your children, on the toys you buy, on their behavior at school. . . . Your first concern is your children's well-being. And there is no reason not to combine breast-feeding with a normal life.

For the first six months, the baby will go through "growth spurts" during which he will suddenly demand more milk. These spurts occur at about six to ten days, three weeks, six weeks, three months, and six months. Your breasts will need two or three days to produce the increased quantity she demands.

It is therefore extremely important to nurse intensively, and above all, not to wean the baby mistakenly, thinking that your milk supply has run dry. If you offer the baby other foods, she will sleep more and nurse less often, just at the time when she needs nursing most. And your milk production will decline for good.

Around six to eight weeks after delivery, some mothers have the impression that their breasts are less full. This simply corresponds to the fact that the breast tissues have adjusted to the larger volume. It does not mean that your supply is declining.

If you have the impression that your baby is often asking for "snacks," he is in fact stimulating your breasts to increase your milk production. On the other hand, these "snacks" can also be a bad habit. If you think that is the case, try to lengthen the time between feedings by fifteen minutes every day, until you reach a more comfortable rhythm.

At the end of two months, in most cases, the breast-feeding routine is well established. You can now go out and leave the baby for several hours, or even a whole day. Your letdown reflex will work without the baby's suction, which allows you to pump your milk much more easily. Most babies are now willing to drink from a bottle without then rejecting the breast. (It is critical to introduce the bottle after nursing is well-established but before the baby gets too attached to the breast. This window of opportunity is at around four to six weeks after birth.)

## If Your Milk Supply Diminishes

Fatigue has a direct impact on milk production. You will have to adopt one of these emergency solutions:

+ Go to bed for a day and a half. Sleep, relax, cut yourself off from the outside world, and put yourself in a bubble with your baby.
+ Get extra help for the older children, as though you were sick.
+ Postpone any planned visits and activities.
+ Drink half a gallon of liquid per day (especially water).

## If the Baby Is Not Putting on Weight

The best remedy is not to supplement with formula.
    Instead, you should:

+ Make sure your nursing position is right (see pages 164 to 168).
+ Dedicate two or three days to the baby during which you will feed him frequently.
+ Wake him up if he sleeps more than six hours.
+ Listen to his gulping. If he stops swallowing, switch breasts. Alternate every ten minutes.
+ Try to nurse in a calm, softly lit environment.
+ If the baby seems to want to nurse only on one side, first offer the side he likes least.

After two or three days, you should have more milk, and the baby will drink more.

## Returning to Work

Going back to work does not mean having to stop breast-feeding. In the United States, 50 percent of mothers who breast-feed while in the hospital are still breast-feeding their baby after six months. Mothers who work can nurse once in the morning, once more when they come home, and again at bedtime. Between feedings, they can pump their milk at the office. During the day, the baby can drink breast milk that has been stored in the refrigerator (but not for more than forty-eight hours). On the weekend, however, the baby must take all of his feeds from the breast. This ensures that if the milk supply is lagging on Friday night, it will be fully restored by Monday morning.

# Weaning

There exists a misconception that weaning is easier during the first month, and that the infant will put up less resistance. It is important to remember, however, that even though a newborn has few means to express himself, he can still feel very frustrated. Weaning should be carried out gently at any age, and never associated with separation or abandonment. That means you should organize yourself so that you do not wean just before a trip or before you go back to work. It should also happen, if possible, when the baby is in good shape—when he doesn't have a cold, or when he is not teething. Take time to cuddle him, and to compensate the link you are cutting with added tenderness.

All it takes to wean is to replace one breast-feeding session—preferably not the one in morning or at bedtime—with a bottle of formula. After a few days, your milk production will diminish. Then another nursing session is replaced, and so on. Your milk supply will diminish and then disappear. Once the baby is fully weaned, your breasts will return to their pre-pregnancy size and shape. You may continue to have a little milk in your breasts for a few more weeks, but that should not be a problem. The longer the period during which you breast-fed (at least five months), the more shapely your breasts will be after weaning.

If your breasts continue to fill at feeding times, pump just enough milk to be comforted, but do not let the baby nurse again, as this will give your body the signal to resume production.

Many women find the emotional aspect of weaning much more difficult than the mechanical side. Weaning signifies the end of the "bubble" period, during which mother and child were in their own world. Breaking off this relationship sometimes is harder to accept than the cutting of the umbilical cord at birth. Share your feelings and worries with a midwife or doula, who can bring you precious moral support during this period.

In the weeks or months that follow the end of breast-feeding, some women can feel one or two small cysts in their breasts. These are simply small nodes that appear in the milk ducts that have not fully drained themselves of milk. Do not touch them or put pressure on them; they will disappear spontaneously after a few months.

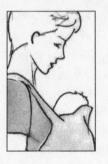

# 16

# The Nursing Mother's Diet

A nursing mother produces 23 to 27 ounces of milk per day, containing 330 milligrams of calcium per quart. This requires an extra energy expenditure of at least 500 calories per day. Good nutrition is therefore just as important for you as it is for your baby.

The quality of breast milk is only affected in extreme cases of deprivation, or by excessive intake of a particular food. But the quantity of milk depends very much on the mother's diet. Food absorbed by a nursing mother not only fulfills her own nutritional needs, which are greater during the postnatal period, but also enables her to produce milk. A woman who does not feed herself properly may still have a healthy baby, but it will be to the detriment of her own health. If you lack sufficient nourishment, your body will make milk production its first priority, and your needs will go unmet. It is just the same as it was during pregnancy, when the nutritional needs of the fetus were satisfied before those of the mother. In fact, the baby, who weighs only a few pounds, will receive nearly 1,000 calories per day in breast milk!

What does it mean to feed yourself properly while nursing? We can compare a breast-feeding mother to a marathon runner—whose race will last twenty-four hours, not four.

# The Basics

Increase your water consumption by one quart per day, so that you are drinking a total of 2.5 to 3 quarts. Nursing women tend to be thirstier anyway, especially during feeding sessions, because part of their water consumption goes directly to milk production. But don't overdo it: too much liquid also can reduce milk production.

Increase your daily caloric intake to 2,500 calories: you can even eat more if you are planning to continue breast-feeding for more than three months (2,800 calories per day). But again, be careful: many nursing mothers are tempted by sweets. Stick to healthy foods instead!

Eat more proteins. The basic rule is to eat 1 gram of protein each day for every pound you weigh.

Spread your caloric intake over five "meals," breakfast, lunch, afternoon snack, dinner, and an extra snack during the evening. Each snack time is also an opportunity to drink water, eat a low-fat dairy product, and a piece of fruit. As your body is continually producing milk, it needs your caloric intake to be regular.

Stay away from tobacco. Nicotine passes directly through breast milk to the baby. If you cannot control yourself, build in a gap of at least an hour between your last cigarette and your next feeding session, so that the nicotine in your system has a chance to decompose at least partially.

Avoid regular consumption of alcohol. Alcohol passes through milk in less than an hour and if the baby consumes it in large quantities it can retard his growth. If you drink an occasional glass of wine or beer, save it for after a feeding session.

Take no medication without first consulting a doctor. Most antibiotics, sulfa drugs, chemical laxatives, and all products containing iodine are contraindicated while you are breast-feeding. Other medications, taken over a long period, can also be dangerous.

Beware of pollutants. Like nicotine, pesticide residue easily passes through mother's milk. If you are nursing, stay away from insecticides (especially in airborne forms such as aerosols or coils). Try to use natural insect repellents such as citronella.

Eat primarily unsaturated fats. Sunflower, corn, rapeseed, and olive oil provide fatty acids that are essential for building the baby's nervous system.

Eat food containing vitamin $B_9$. In Western countries, the only vitamin really lacking in women's diets is vitamin $B_9$ (folic acid). Birth control pills accentuate a woman's vitamin $B_9$ deficit, and may also contribute to a vitamin $B_6$ deficiency. During pregnancy, folic acid is vital to the development of the baby's nervous system. Nursing mothers are well advised to continue taking their prenatal vitamins. Folic acid also can be found abundantly in asparagus, cabbage, corn, chickpeas, and spinach. Many other foods, such as wheat and orange juice, have been enriched with folic acid. Check the package labels.

Take zinc supplements. According to a British study, pregnant and nursing women also often lack zinc. They should consume 15 to 20 milligrams per day. Zinc is found in eggs, meat, whole flour, and oats.

Consume 1,200 milligrams of calcium per day. A balanced diet only provides 800 to 1,000 milligrams of calcium daily. Because nursing mothers need 1,200 milligrams, a calcium supplement will probably be necessary. Calcium needs can also be partly met from dairy products, raw vegetables, almonds, and hazelnuts.

Do not rush to buy vitamin A supplements. People often talk about vitamin A supplements for nursing mothers, because their daily need rises from 1,000 milligrams to 1,300 milligrams. It is true that if the woman had a vitamin A deficiency during pregnancy, this problem may worsen after childbirth. But anyone who eats enough carrots, vegetables, butter, fish, and meat will absorb enough vitamin A.

We hear a lot about foods that can irritate the baby—turnips, celery, watercress, citrus fruits, onions, cabbage, spices, leeks, cauliflower—by giving him gas or changing the taste of his mother's milk. For example, some people say that garlic increases milk production; others say it gives the baby gas. There is no universal rule. Moreover, different cultures prefer foods that others consider to be "bad" for nursing mothers. Each baby reacts differently to the foods his mother consumes. If your baby is particularly disturbed one day, try to remember what you have eaten in the past twenty-four hours. If one food seems suspect, eliminate it from your diet for a while.

When nursing, observe your baby so you can eliminate from your own diet any food that seems to bother him.

There exist nutritional supplements that are said to increase milk production. Their effects have not been proven scientifically, but they have a placebo (psychological) effect. Be careful, some of these supplements have a very high sugar content, and are therefore high in calories. Also, many midwives will tell you that fennel and beer increase milk production, and that parsley stops it.

## Additional Resources

La Leche League International
P.O. Box 4079
1400 N. Meacham Rd.
Schaumburg, IL 60173
800-La Leche
ww.lalecheleague.org

Nursing Mothers' Counsel (NMC)
P.O. Box 50063
Palo Alto, CA 94303
Referral Line: 415-386-2229

International Lactation Consultants' Association
4101 Lake Boone Trail
Raleigh, NC 27602
919-787-5181
*ilca@erols.com*

*The Art of Successful Breastfeeding: A Mother's Guide* (Video)
The Vancouver Breastfeeding Center
604-875-5017
*millerb@direct.ca*

*The Womanly Art of Breastfeeding*
The La Leche League
800-La-Leche

# IV

# Emotional Reactions to Childbirth

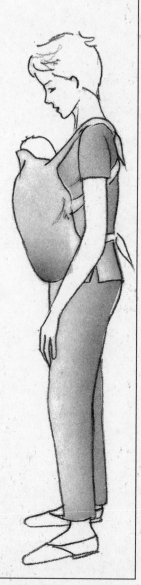

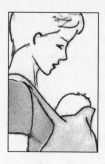

# 17

# The First Days

## A Time of Change

We all know how intimately the mind is linked to the body. Emotions can have physical manifestations—for example, stress increases blood pressure. Likewise, physical problems can have emotional repercussions—pain causes mental fatigue. So it is understandable that childbirth, the greatest physical transformation that a woman can undergo, will affect the mind. The gradual transformations of pregnancy that took place over nine months will reverse themselves in just a few hours; most notably the body's hormonal equilibrium will radically shift. And since hormones are the critical link between the mind and the body, this violent disruption of hormonal production is bound to cause an emotional reaction.

A new mother's mind needs more than a few days to recover from this major event and find a new balance. Many people do not realize that the days immediately following childbirth are a very important period of psychic transition as well as physical healing. A woman's body will return to its pre-pregnant state over the coming weeks, but her "head" may not always follow quite at the same rate. She may have moments of hypersensitivity, worry, and even anxiety. Her dreams will be more intense, sometimes even bizarre. How well she copes with this greater emotional vulnerability depends in large part on her how secure she feels about her new role as a mother, her psychological past, her relationship with her partner, and her place in the world.

According to Dr. James Hamilton, a pioneer in the study of postnatal depression, a mother's emotional reactions evolve during the postpartum period.

The first two or three days, the new mother goes through a "latent phase." Her needs are simple: to eat and sleep. She may appear passive and acquiescent, as if overcome by events. Often she is mentally reviewing over and over again the details of her labor and delivery.

From the third to the eleventh days, the new mother appears more independent and self-sufficient, taking her own initiatives. Little by little, she establishes a routine with her baby and begins to manage her new situation. But her hormone levels are at their lowest point now and she is entering an emotional "danger" zone of negative reactions to the birth. Doubts and worries begin to surface. She may mourn her "dream baby," the child she has imagined for the past nine months who looks nothing like the real baby in her arms. This is her moment of greatest vulnerability when the slightest misplaced word takes on giant proportions. The physical symptoms of this troubled period are predominantly tears and mood swings, commonly known as the "baby blues."

From the eleventh day onwards, through the first six weeks, the "baby blues" are over, but a mother may still feel "depressed" due to her tiredness, physical or emotional discomfort. This also is the point at which the friends and family who appeared so enthusiastic during the first days after the baby's birth now drift away—just when she needs the most support. She may begin to feel cut off from the adult world, or sometimes even "suffocated" by the baby. For one woman in ten, these negative feelings worsen steadily and become a psychiatric illness known as "postnatal depression."

Between the second and fourth months after childbirth, a new routine is established, and the new mother usually feels more confident and less vulnerable. The baby is learning to sleep on her own and seems more easily satisfied. But fatigue and loneliness are still very much a reality: four in ten cases of postnatal depression begin at this stage.

## Your First Encounter with the Baby

At first, mother and baby try to elicit responses from one another. It's a period of "mutual seduction." The mother spontaneously uses a softer, more melodious tone of voice—and the baby responds by turning his head towards her. As the baby searches for his mother's nipple, the mother knows she can fulfill his need, and thus feels valuable and wanted. Within a few weeks the baby will show his contentment—he gurgles, smiles, and looks his mother straight in the eye. She melts with happiness.

The famous British pediatrician and psychologist Donald Winnicott studied at length the new mother's state of hypersensitivity during pregnancy and in the few weeks following childbirth. He labeled this frame of mind "primary maternal preoccupation" and explained it as a natural phenomenon that allows a mother to be more attuned to her child, thus better able to care for him.

Winnicott also noticed that a woman's subconscious seems to be more present at this time: old memories come flooding back. He spoke even of an "ordinary madness" in new mothers, a kind of regression into the past that permits a mother to identify deeply with her newborn and to understand his needs almost instinctively.

Countless studies of the bonding process between mother and infant show that this mechanism is very complex. A mother's interest in her baby does not necessarily immediately include love—quite the contrary, more than 40 percent of new mothers admit to feelings of indifference and even hostility towards their baby. Often they are concerned that these emotions are abnormal because they fly against traditional images of "happy motherhood." So they tend to hide their feelings, even from their partners, sometimes fearing that something will happen to their baby if they do not display enough maternal love.

## Mixed Feelings

Negative thoughts, anxieties, and doubts are very common among new mothers. Here are some examples of feelings many mothers have experienced after childbirth:

### Numbness, Indifference

Some mothers see the newborn as a complete stranger. The tremendous rush of maternal love they expected to feel simply did not materialize. This baby is so different from the baby they had dreamt about for nine months! The emptiness in their belly, which had been so full during pregnancy, can sometimes be accompanied by a similar emptiness in the heart.

### An Emotional Overinvestment

In contrast, some mothers may become completely absorbed by the baby and ignore everything else. They act a bit as they would with a new lover. They are alert, high-strung, quick to misconstrue any comment about the baby (he's too fat, not fat enough, he looks like his father). This state of nervous tension causes them to swing between exhilaration and despair.

### A Fear of Losing One's Self

Life now becomes organized around the baby, who seems always to come first. Friends and family focus all of their attention on the baby. Some women react as though they are being "devoured" by this little creature. They may look to the baby for signs of gratitude for the "sacrifice" that they are making. If he happens not to react as expected—he does not open his eyes or gurgle because he is drowsy, cries or refuses to nurse—his mother may misinterpret such insignificant reactions and feel further discouragement.

### A Loss of Status

During her pregnancy, a future mother is often the center of attention. After giving birth, she suddenly reverts to being an ordinary woman—in a sense losing her "aura." This change in status can be extremely disorienting to some women who have a hard time no longer being the star. In other cultures, motherhood is a consecration, the crowning achievement of womanhood. In ours, being a mother is only one in a series of possible choices, and even excludes us from some of the other options. Some women might even feel that they are in competition with their own child, especially if they did not receive enough attention when they were young girls.

## Anxiety

Young mothers, particularly those giving birth for the first time, are often troubled by innumerable doubts. They may worry about the baby's health, even if it is excellent. They may fear that they will not be able to protect this fragile creature. They may doubt their aptitude at being a "good mother;" they may feel incompetent or overwhelmed by events. They may wonder if their partner can be a good and affectionate father, who will adequately provide for the family's financial and emotional needs. They may be apprehensive about returning to work. And they may worry about recovering their intimacy with their spouse.

New mothers who have a history of miscarriages, premature births, or infertility usually are more anxious during pregnancy. They also tend to remain anxious after giving birth, which can make their first contacts with the baby somewhat tense.

## Disappointment

If the delivery takes an unforeseen turn (emergency cesarean, forceps, even anesthesia if the woman thought that she would not need any), the mother may feel very discouraged. Disappointment may also overcome happiness if the baby is a different sex than was hoped for, or if the baby's physical appearance is offensive to his mother. Many new parents do not realize that the babies we see in advertisements are already a few months old, so they are surprised to see this tiny, "wrinkled" creature that may look like an alien or an old man. Some mothers turn disappointment into guilt and blame themselves for what they perceive as a failure. Others may turn their back on the baby, or pay attention to him only if others are looking on.

## Mourning the "Dream Baby"

This is a term used by psychologists to explain the melancholy many mothers feel after childbirth. During her pregnancy, a woman carries her baby not only in her womb but also in her heart and in her mind. All future mothers fantasize about their baby-to-be. After delivery, the infant is in an isolette beside her but no longer in the womb; the secret, intimate presence has disappeared. The real baby, who is inevitably different than the imagined one, is either a wonderful surprise or a disappointment, particularly if his sex or appearance doesn't coincide with his parents' expectations. The profound sadness that some mothers feel just after giving birth is in fact mourning for their "dream baby." Even if a mother does not feel deep grief, there inevitably will be moments when she wishes that she could "zip him back in" to feel the special closeness of pregnancy.

It takes time for a mother to overcome these doubts and fears, and to "fall in love" with her baby—from a few days to several weeks. Ideally, she will need a calm and supportive atmosphere in order to focus on building her relationship with the baby. Unfortunately, many women do not have such a luxury and return home to face increased housekeeping and child-care duties, financial worries, or a tense relationship with their partner. Organizing the return home well before the birth (see tips on pages 100 to 104) and learning how to handle stress (see pages 226 to 229) can help a new mother find the time necessary for this critical process. Furthermore, specialized help is always available—the hard part is finding the courage to ask. Sometimes, just one meeting with a nurse-midwife trained in psychology or a psychotherapist is enough to help an anxious mother get "back on track."

It is comforting to remember that each one of us has a deep, basic need to go beyond our own self-love and to care for someone more vulnerable, to learn to love unconditionally. When any initial doubts and negative emotions begin to fade, when we get used to our new role as mothers, this love will blossom. Nearly all mothers fall deeply and passionately in love with their children.

## Communicating with the Newborn

Today, communicating with our child starts well before birth. Sonograms, fetal medicine, fertility treatments, and many of the popular childbirth preparation methods have all transformed the mother-child relationship into something very concrete long before they actually see each other. Pregnant mothers have never taken such good care of themselves, and thus, indirectly, of the baby growing inside them. Future mothers now speak to their babies in utero or play music. Many parents start their baby album with a sonogram picture. All this prenatal information can be comforting . . . or very discomforting if a health problem arises or if the baby's sex is not what was desired.

When the baby is born, he is welcomed as a full-fledged human being. The psychology of the newborn is a recognized field of special-

## SINGLE MOTHERS

According to many midwives, single mothers often need more time to adapt and bond with their new babies than do mothers who are in a stable relationship. There are many possible explanations for this:

- For many couples, having a baby represents a milestone, an accomplishment that validates the couple. For a single mother, a child may be the reminder of a failed relationship, or of a passion that did not last.
- A single mother who has a baby in the hopes of gaining a companion may suddenly realize that she will have to wait a lot longer than she had anticipated before he reaches maturity. Often, the desire for pregnancy is impulsive, almost "carnal." Maternal instinct, however, is something completely different—a mixture of tenderness and a sense of responsibility.
- Once the baby is born, a single mother may feel overwhelmed by the challenge of raising a child alone. Single mothers may have serious financial and material concerns that cause stress and tension to cloud their first interactions with the baby.

Despite these initial difficulties, there is no reason why a single mother cannot go on to have just as positive a postnatal experience as a woman who is in a steady relationship.

ization. A growing number of hospitals offer neonatal psychiatry. And yet, we still use the same basic tools to communicate with our babies as our ancestors did thousands of years ago: touch, sight, and voice.

From the baby's perspective, communication while in the womb primarily happened through the placenta, but also through touch and sound if his mother stroked her belly or spoke to him. Once he is born, he also uses sight and smell. Numerous studies demonstrate that the newborn quickly learns to recognize the smell of his mother's milk. The newborn has a field of vision of only 5½ inches, which corresponds to the distance between his face and his mother's when he is at the breast. This explains why newborns seem to stare intently at their mothers while nursing: it's actually one of the few times they get a clear picture that really interests them!

The skin is an effective way of communicating because it is in contact with the baby's nervous system, which in turn acts on his respira-

## A FEW TIPS

- Don't be too rigid. There are no hard and fast rules—especially not to be found in books.
- Have faith in your intuition and maternal instinct.
- Don't compare your baby to other babies, even to his brothers or sisters.
- Don't look for your flaws in your baby; this means inventing personality traits that do not exist and will interfere with your ability to "listen" to his needs.
- Don't use food as a means of communication: mothers often judge their child's personality by his eating habits. This can become an obsession.

tory and vital organs. During labor, it has been shown that uterine contractions act like a deep massage, an important source of tactile stimulation for the baby. After his birth, the baby needs to be held, carried, caressed. Fortunately, people no longer say a baby is "spoiled" if it spends too much time in our arms. In fact, research shows that the production of certain antibodies that help the baby resist infection is stimulated by direct contact between mother and infant. While this immune resistance is less strong than that provided by breast milk, it is an important source for babies who are not breast-fed.

An excellent way to implement this advice is through baby massage. Many maternity centers teach this, and massage techniques can also be found in books and videos. However, mothers generally do not need to be taught a special technique to stroke their baby. On the contrary, concentrating on a particular "method" can distract a mother from listening to the baby's responses instead of simply remembering the advice of Dr. Frédéric Leboyer, one of the fathers of "natural childbirth": the hands that hold should speak the language of womb so as to soften the onslaught of this strange and incomprehensible world. Constant physical contact with the baby also is extremely beneficial to the mother, as it sustains the production of prolactin, the "maternal instinct hormone."

A mother's voice has a magical effect. Even if a baby does not understand the content of the words spoken to him, he will respond to the tone of voice used. This is why it is extremely important to speak to your baby, to explain what is happening and what you are doing to him (especially if it's painful), and to share your concerns when they pertain to him. When a mother releases tension by sharing her worries with her baby, he will respond by relaxing. The more talk a baby infant hears around him, the more easily he will begin to undertake some vocal communication himself (this does not mean, however, that you have to talk all the time; a baby also needs some calm and silence).

## Caring for the Baby

In the past, little girls grew up surrounded by several generations. Throughout their childhood, they heard their grandmothers, aunts, and cousins giving advice on child care. They were in frequent contact with nursing mothers and infants and they often helped with the babies.

Today, with the exception of eldest children in large families, girls have little contact with babies beyond a little baby-sitting when they are teenagers. In our culture, the young live with the young; the old with the old. Couples often live together for long periods of time before having children. Fathers today are even less prepared than future mothers, yet they are expected to share fully in child-care responsibilities. Worse, if we delay childbirth into our thirties, our own mothers seem to have forgotten everything ("that was a long time ago, dear") or claim that things are so different now that they cannot help us. And if we have our children early, our mothers either live too far away or are too busy with their own careers. For many young mothers, the only chance to have some practice time under professional guidance will be the two days or so they will spend in the hospital (interestingly, surveys show that many new mothers judge the quality of their hospital stay by the quantity of information and support they receive from the maternity nurses who give them their first lessons in caring for the newborn).

Because there are often too few maternity nurses to go around, they may always seem too busy. But if asked for help, they generally are more than willing to assist new mothers. Unfortunately, many women don't dare ask for help because the hospital environment is too intimidating. It is important to remember that the primary responsibility of the nursing team is to help you get started in the new challenge of motherhood. Insist that the nurses allow you to practice caring for the baby under their supervision. Ask them to correct you or to show you a better way. Ask them to give you answers and suggestions.

A good place to start is a very simple activity: holding your child. Ask the nurse to place the baby properly in your arms. A baby isn't fragile. Whichever position you choose, be sure that you are supporting his pelvis, and let him look at you unencumbered.

While in the hospital, don't hesitate to ask for advice from second- or third-time mothers. They generally will be delighted to share their knowledge about things that seem old hat to them now!

## The Never-ending Story
## of Childbirth

In the days following childbirth, women tend to think over every minute of their delivery. As soon as they are asked, "How did it go?" new mothers will happily provide a lengthy account of the birth. Even years later, women are always happy to recount their experience— although with time, a "happy amnesia" will tend to blot out the more difficult passages, unless they were particularly painful or traumatic. But in the hours and days following the birth, some women may feel frustrated if they cannot remember its every detail. This sense of dissatisfaction may lead to anger toward the medical team or to a sense that something "went wrong" with the birth. In such cases, it is useful to write down as many details as possible which can be reviewed later when the mother has come out of the state of emotional upheaval and oversensitivity that follows childbirth.

These days, new mothers tend to be under the influence of three myths:

**"Childbirth is an end in itself."** The media, most pregnancy books, and even some childbirth instructors describe labor and delivery as a finality. Pregnancy is a slow crescendo, which reaches its climax in the birth process. What happens afterwards is either not described or treated only summarily. After the birth, everyone's attention shifts to the baby. Yet, the birth is only one step in the maternal process! A woman's body will undergo as many changes in the nine months following childbirth as it did during pregnancy. If the postnatal period received the preparation and attention of pregnancy and the birth itself, fewer women would complain that they were "caught completely unaware."

**"Childbirth is a rite of passage."** In the past, women were grateful to be alive after having given birth. Today, they view the delivery as a seminal event in their lives, a form of enlightenment. They read several pregnancy books, take preparation classes, and spend hours questioning friends. But if things don't happen as expected, the disappointed will be bitter. Everyone wants the birth to "go well," but "well" for the mother may be different from "well" for the doctor. While most women understand the necessity of medical intervention, some see it as a violation. An emergency cesarean section, use of forceps, or even recourse to anesthesia or an epidural when a natural delivery was planned, can all be experienced as a failure by the mother who was hoping for a "perfect birth." She may feel that something was denied her, that she did not succeed in her task.

**"A good start is necessary to a good life."** During their pregnancies, women worry that stressful events (a death in the family, an accident, problems at work) will cause them anxiety and harm the "perfect" environment they want to create for the fetus. In the same way, a mother also can feel a strong sense of guilt or regret if she thinks that her child will be marked for life by a bad delivery. This sense of failure is often the product of her unreasonable expectations. Every well-prepared delivery is a positive experience, whether it is entirely natural or requiring medical intervention.

A child's emotional development is an evolutionary process, marked more by a succession of influences than by specific events. Therefore, one event in a baby's early life will have a serious impact on his personality only if it repeats itself. The process evolves continuously: there is always the chance to "catch up," and to correct previous errors.

Fortunately, most women have positive memories of their birth experiences. We tend to forget the difficult moments: it's nature's way of ensuring that women will have more than one baby!

# Special Cases

## A Premature Baby

"Medically induced" prematurity is on the rise due to an increase in the number of multiple pregnancies (primarily from fertility treatments) and in the number of induced births (when the baby is not growing properly or if the mother's health is threatened such as in cases of hypertension). In any given large hospital, about 30 percent of premature births are linked to twins, triplets, and other multiple births. Almost half of all twins (49 percent) are born early, while 97 percent of triplets and 100 percent of quadruplets are born prematurely. Induced births have risen 20 percent in the past fifteen years.

When a baby is taken away right after birth for neonatal care, some mothers may wonder if they would not be better off not seeing their child until he has recovered. They are, consciously or not, guarding against becoming too emotionally attached to a baby in case the outcome is not a happy one. But nevertheless, a newborn in the incubator needs contact with his mother right from the start.

Other mothers may feel strong guilt about not having bonded with their baby right from the start. If the mother must return home without the baby, or with only one of two twins, she will face the additional, exhausting task of shuttling back and forth to the hospital until the baby comes home.

In situations where highly specialized care is required, a mother can be made to feel incompetent and useless. The hospital environment lacks intimacy and almost inevitably puts her in a position of inferiority. Fortunately, a growing number of hospitals provide neonatal specialists trained in communicating with the baby's parents and helping them through this difficult time.

Our generation has been greatly influenced by Dr. Leboyer's work on nonviolent birth and on the importance of immediate contact between mother and newborn. But recent scientific research has shown that a separation between mother and newborn does not prevent the mother from loving her child. If they must wait several days finally to meet, there will be no long-term repercussions on the child's development, provided that she is raised in a loving and stable environment.

Many studies have shown that with babies who were born with serious complications any developmental lag a baby may have at one year of age will be completely overcome by the time she turns ten, if he grows up in a positive and supportive environment.

## A Sick Baby

The enormous advances of the past two decades in prenatal diagnosis techniques mean that it is now rare to discover an illness or a serious congenital defect only at the moment of the baby's birth. But the media coverage of these medical breakthroughs has led many of us to believe in the omnipotence of medicine—and made it very difficult to accept a problem. Any defect, no matter how minor to the scientific community, will never be insignificant to a parent.

If the mother is not prepared for a serious disorder in her child, her first impulse may be to escape, to flee her "deficient" child. This desire to flee may extend to a death wish. In cases where the baby is seriously ill or handicapped, doctors and midwives often hear the words: "I don't want to see him; why should I become attached to him if he is going to die?" or "If he is going to be handicapped, I'd prefer that he died." This reaction is not meant for the baby whom the mother has been carrying in her heart and in her womb for the past nine months, but for the "impostor" she sees now, covered in tubes and surrounded by the Plexiglas of an incubator. The desire to flee and abandon the sick infant usually is felt most strongly while the mother is in the maternity ward, surrounded by happy mothers with healthy babies.

An abnormal infant therefore must be "adopted" by his family. It is a difficult and lengthy process, because it also involves mourning the end of a dream, and accepting bitter disappointment. The most difficult task for the mother of an abnormal or seriously unhealthy baby is to reconcile herself with the feeling of having failed. She may interpret the deformity or illness in her child as a punishment, a form of "divine retribution" for past acts. Or she may feel guilty for not having taken greater care during her pregnancy.

The parents of a handicapped baby are faced with four challenges to overcome:

1. **Disappointment**. The child's handicap shatters the picture they had imagined of their new life as a family.
2. **Tension within the couple**. Each partner seeks to determine what was responsible for the mishap: what could they have done to deserve such a child? They begin to doubt their capacity to bring a healthy child into the world.
3. **Anger**. In order to foster a loving relationship with their handicapped child, they must overcome this anger.
4. **Shame and resentment**. This is what the couple feels toward their extended family and friends who have normal children.

## Reactions Toward the Medical Team

Parents also tend to accuse the doctors of incompetence even if nothing medical could have been done to prevent the defect. But it is important to remember that doctors and nurses also suffer from a feeling of impotence, not knowing what to say or do. Many times the news is broken in a clumsy fashion: sometimes a doctor or nurse will overinform the parents, by saying too much at once. A wish to protect the parents may lead to exaggerating optimism or pessimism. If there already exists tension or communication problems between the parents and the medical team, this can complicate the announcement of a problem. In all cases, parents should try to talk only with the doctors and midwives who are closely involved with the situation. Hopefully, the caregivers will explain the situation clearly and simply, and also will help the parents formulate the explanations they will be giving to family and friends. Any serious obstetric event such as a severe birth defect or a stillbirth should be followed by a doctor's visit in order to analyze the situation. This consultation is also important to reassure the parents about any future pregnancies.

The mother of a baby with complications at birth needs to be able to speak with experts who can give her coherent and correct information. She often needs to talk about the sequence of events, especially if the delivery was difficult or traumatic. Fortunately, medical personnel are now better trained to listen and to explain, rather than simply provide empty reassurances. Neonatal units often include a staff psychologist who can help the mother overcome the ordeal of giving birth to a handicapped or sick child. And obstetricians can recommend therapists who will support the mother emotionally once she has brought the baby home.

## "Baby Blues"

Some 70 to 80 percent of new mothers experience a harmless form of depression between the third and the eleventh day after giving birth. This state of emotional upheaval generally lasts two to seven days. It should not be confused with postnatal depression, which lasts longer, and which we will discuss further on in this section.

The symptoms of the "baby blues" are:

◆ Frequent tears for apparently minor reasons.
◆ Mood swings.
◆ Irritability and hypersensitivity to criticism.
◆ Difficulty in concentrating.
◆ Anxiety about one's ability to look after the baby.
◆ Difficulties in bonding with the newborn.
◆ Feelings of discouragement or vulnerability.
◆ Restless sleep patterns.

A new mother can feel euphoric one minute and then the next minute melt into a pool of tears. These are tears of emotion and not of grief, as is the case with a true postnatal depression. It also is quite normal for a new mother to continue having mood swings for several weeks even after she has passed through the "blues" stage.

**"Baby blues" affect women of all socioeconomic levels, no matter what their relationship with their partner, and no matter what their childbirth experience has been. Even fathers can experience a sort of "baby blues."**

"Baby blues" can affect women who gave birth at home just as they affect those who delivered in a hospital. However, tears are easier to hide at home. They often punctuate a difficult moment: when the episiotomy starts to heal and it pulls on the stitches; when the baby goes through a growth spurt and seems to constantly want more attention. For many women who give birth in a hospital, the tears start the day they return home.

It is interesting to note that in cases of premature birth, "baby blues" don't start until the baby is reunited with his mother, sometimes even as late as two months after the birth. This phenomenon is therefore highly complex. It is linked not only to the physical effects of childbirth, but also to the mother-child relationship and to the emotions brought on by the arrival of a baby.

## Causes

### *Hormones*
During pregnancy, the placenta acts as lung, digestive tract, and kidney for the fetus. It also secretes the hormones (notably estrogen and

progesterone) necessary for the normal development of the pregnancy. Progesterone diminishes the production of monoamine oxidase (MAO), a substance that acts upon the emotional center of the brain to produce depressive reactions (a healthy body must produce "downers" as well as "uppers" to keep emotions in balance). During pregnancy, the level of progesterone is 30 to 50 times higher than normal, which explains the feeling of euphoria experienced by many expectant mothers, particularly during the second trimester.

When the placenta is expelled at the end of childbirth, hormone levels fall abruptly over the course of a few hours—as opposed to their slow rise over the nine months of pregnancy. This is a major shock for the body that can severely affect the hypothalamus, the lower part of the brain that controls the menstrual clock, the emotions, the body's weight, and day/night rhythms. The situation is further unsettled by the fact that the ovaries, which have been asleep for nine months, may have a hard time getting back into their old hormone production role. On top of this, every new mother's body releases prolactin, the "milk supply hormone," which tends to inhibit the normal production of estrogen and progesterone whether the woman breast-feeds or not. This inhibiting effect can last for more than two months.

Thus hormonal disturbance is considerable—and emotional repercussions are the result.

### Fatigue

Fatigue brings on depression. Most mothers are exhausted after delivering a baby. If their labor was long, they probably missed a night's sleep. They probably arrived at the hospital already tired from weeks of interrupted nights during the last month of pregnancy. Added to the physical fatigue is the nervous tension of giving birth, the suffering, and the worry. Afterward, the physical results of childbirth, the pain of an episiotomy, hemorrhoids, or the scar of a cesarean section also inhibit sleep. Hospital wards rarely provide a restful environment in which to recuperate. And, toward the third day after delivery, the arrival of milk in the breasts is also tiring.

### Uncertainty and Regrets

The arrival of a baby can unleash a crisis of self-confidence. Even if the new mother thinks she has "prepared" for the birth, by reading and asking advice, she is surprised by the baby's apparent vulnerability. The mother is thrown off track by the number of new things she has to know, and by how little direction her baby gives her. In a medical environment, surrounded by specialists, she forgets that her maternal instinct and common sense are the best guides. The maternal feeling, so new to her, is fragile: "It's not normal. Yesterday he opened his eyes and drank, but he has been sleeping nonstop since yesterday evening." She doubts her ability to satisfy her baby. All of this constitutes a shock for the woman who until now felt that she was in charge of her own life.

The feeling of powerlessness can be aggravated if the childbirth was a difficult one, and if the sequence of events didn't happen as she had anticipated. We have seen that many women feel they have "failed" in childbirth if they had to undergo an emergency cesarean section, if forceps were used, or even if they ended up using anesthesia, when they had expected to be able to master their own pain.

Women don't usually realize the extent to which regret is one of the principal emotions felt after childbirth. They miss their full, fertile belly, which now is empty, or they are disappointed if the father is not behaving as they had hoped he would. They have also lost their status as a little girl, and must now become a responsible mother, taking their turn to pay attention to another.

### Losing the Status of Pregnancy

During the first days after childbirth, many women miss the "simplicity" of their pregnant days. Before the baby arrived, they had few responsibilities and benefited from enormous amounts of attention. While pregnant, they were pampered, taken care of, watched over by doctors, treated as the "intermediary" between the baby they carried and the outside world. During delivery, they were the center of the universe. Suddenly, all the attention has shifted to the baby. And it is not easy to give up one's role as the star! Friends and relatives run straight to the cradle without asking how the mother is doing. Many women have waited months, sometimes years, only to find their womb empty and themselves ignored. Even the medical staff seems to be no longer interested in the mother, except for the necessary medical procedures, while the baby entrances the whole world. For other women, the hardest part is being relegated to a single role, that of mother.

This psychological fragility is often accentuated by the disappointment that most women feel in regard to their own bodies. They would like to recover and to quickly regain their lost equilibrium. But it takes months to do that. They must accept that their bodies will never be the same, that a mother's body has a new appearance, and that it fulfills new functions.

### *The Hospital Environment*

The hospital is usually not a restful place: constant footsteps, nurses coming at all hours to check your vitals, the cleaning staff who enter without knocking, the elevator doors, the breakfast carts, the cries of babies—not to mention phone calls and visitors. If the new mother is sharing a room, she can be sure that her roommate's baby probably will not be on the same feeding schedule as her own. The mother's relationship with midwives, doctors, and nurses may be tense, especially while the she is in a hypersensitive state.

It is also important to know that tears are "contagious." Seeing one's roommate cry is all it takes to provoke one's own tears. And some young nurses feel uncomfortable seeing older women crying. Medical staff may unwittingly give contradictory answers to the same question, or appear to underestimate a problem. The slightest word from them may have an enormous impact. For this reason, maternity floor personnel should be particularly careful about what they say. If a nurse lets slip that the baby cries too much, or has a bad temper, the new mother may overreact dramatically.

A woman can find the hospital atmosphere so stressful that she fights back the baby blues there and melts down when she gets home! But do not forget that while you are in the hospital you are surrounded by specialists who are there to help you.

## Handling the "Baby Blues"

Because the "baby blues" is not an illness, it can be "treated" with rest and support. More and more hospitals are now offering psychologists' services. Don't hesitate to ask to meet one if you wish to speak calmly with someone professional. The father can also play a vital role by limiting the number of visitors you receive while you are in the hospital. In any case, there's no point worrying too much—the "baby blues" are always temporary. (If the tears continue beyond two weeks after delivery, it may be a case of depression and this is treated fully in Chapter 19.) On the contrary, this state of acute sensitivity helps the mother become attuned to her baby and establish the close mother-infant contact.

# BABY BLUES

## Homeopathy

- For general well-being: take 4 granules China 4C in the morning, 4 granules Ambra Grisea 7C before bed.
- If you are feeling indifferent or numb: take 1 initial dose of Natrum Muriacum 15C, and then 3 granules 9C every morning.
- If you are sad, or become sadder as people try to console you: take 1 dose Sepia 15C, and then 3 granules 9C every morning.
- If the "blues" are mainly due to fatigue from delivery (especially after a hemorrhage): take China 5C twice a day.
- If you feel exhausted and empty: take Phosphoricum Acidum 9C twice a day.

## Herbal Remedies

- The following infusion will help calm the spirit: Raspberry Leaf tea with equal quantities of either Peppermint or Spearmint.
- Another infusion to help restore emotional balance is made with Burdock, Blessed Thistle, and Orange Peel.

## Aromatherapy

- Take 1 drop essential oil of Cinnamon and 1 drop essential oil of Ravensar (Ravensare Aromatica) on a sugar cube three times a day. Cinnamon is a stimulant and is effective when physical fatigue affects the psyche. Ravensar is also an excellent combatant of fatigue and exhaustion. Essential oil of Ravensar also can be used to massage the nape of the neck.
- Essential oil of Rose also is recommended to fight the baby blues.
- Herbalists also recommend burning a mix of essential oils of Orange, Bergamot, Mandarin, Neroli, Geranium, and Rose in a diffuser or making a 6 percent blend of these oils to use in the bath.
- Among the Bach Flower Remedies, the Rescue mixture, composed of Star of Bethlehem, Helianthemum, Clematis, Prunus, and Impatience is particularly effective. A few drops should be squirted under the tongue several times a day.

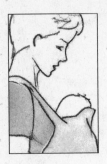

# 18

# Emotional Reactions of the First Few Months

In the weeks after childbirth, most new mothers will at some point feel extremely tired, depressed, overwhelmed, or drained of energy. One woman in ten will suffer from an emotional reaction sufficiently strong to justify seeking medical or psychiatric treatment. How can we distinguish between the various emotional reactions of childbirth? How do we know if medical help is necessary? What kinds of treatments are available?

In 1858, a French physician, Dr. L. V. Marcé, was the first to study the emotional difficulties brought on by childbirth in a scientific way. But it was not until nearly a hundred years later, when doctors finally had mastered postnatal infections (until 1950, the leading cause of death among childbearing women), that researchers could concentrate on this topic. Despite the fact that women have suffered from postnatal depression for generations, most of the information you will find in this chapter dates from the last twenty years. Perinatal psychology is a recent science, which explains in part why today there are so many contradictory theories. The following is an overview that may help clarify the issues.

## Different Types of Postnatal Distress

It is important to understand the difference between the different types of postnatal reactions.

**The baby blues**. This is a transient, short-term state of depression principally of hormonal origin, clearly identified by the symptoms described on pages 210 to 211. However, more serious emotional problems are sometimes mistaken for a simple case of "baby blues," leading new mothers, and their doctors, to underestimate the problem.

**A number of depressive reactions** are often caused by exhaustion, and these are generally remedied by more sleep, better nutrition or nutritional supplements, support and assistance with household chores, recreation, or a few sessions with a psychotherapist.

**Postnatal depression**. This really should be called "maternal depression," because it's not strictly limited to the postnatal period. This is a psychiatric illness that requires both prescription medication and/or psychotherapy.

**Puerperal psychosis**. This is an extreme form of postnatal depression that requires immediate hospitalization, with symptoms including hallucinations, extreme confusion, and rejection of the baby.

The last three categories of emotional reactions differ from simple "baby blues" in terms of their appearance, their duration, their symptoms, and their treatment (see the chart on page 230). But we have heard so frequently that a bout of baby blues is normal that we tend to believe that a more lasting feeling of depression is only a heavy form of the "blues" that will disappear with time. If women only knew how to identify their symptoms more accurately, they probably would seek professional help much sooner.

## Overcoming Postpartum Distress

Most future mothers do not realize that they will go through several months of emotional ups and downs after the birth of their child. There will be moments of intense happiness and joy, moments of wonderful peace and tranquility, as well as moments of near depression when she will feel exhausted, overwhelmed, frustrated, or incompetent.

## The Causes

Most of the time, these negative feelings are related to three factors—hormonal upheaval, fatigue, and the constraints of a new life.

### Hormonal upheaval

As we have seen, the amount of progesterone and estrogen in a woman near the end of her pregnancy is thirty to fifty times higher than normal. In less than three days, these levels will plummet to nearly zero. When the progesterone count (which has been acting as an antidepressant for nine months) falls so rapidly, it can cause the equivalent of an "emotional earthquake" in the body. Each woman will cope differently with this violent change, depending on her circumstances, her emotional strength, and the support that she receives from her family and friends.

### Fatigue

Every new mother suffers to some extent from lack of sleep. The emotional repercussions are well known: irritability, oversensitivity, and the feeling of "I'm not going to make it" that quickly translates into anger at her baby, her family, and herself.

### Constraints of a New Life

Some people still think that a woman who stays home "has nothing to do" when in fact a new mother must not only recover from the enormous physical upheaval that is childbirth, but also completely restructure her life and habits around the baby. This transformation is often difficult to make. Being more sensitive than normal, a new mother may rapidly feel "overtaken by events." The slightest criticism from those around her will not help matters.

There are also a number of secondary causes that can lead to mild depression. These include the following.

### Physical Causes

+ **Pain,** due to such physical problems as a displaced coccyx, difficulties in breast-feeding, urinary incontinence, hemorrhoids, or varicose veins, will not only prevent a woman from sleeping properly, they can also be debilitating for the body and provoke asthenia (the medical term for fatigue). Fortunately, all of these problems can be cured.

The relationship between physical pain, fatigue, and depression is an important topic that is currently being studied by researchers. Women tend to assign their emotional suffering to a part of their body that is already weak, very often the back. Some specialists think that women make this transposition because they dare not appear to be "unhappy mothers." Ironically, we have the right to be tired or sore, but not sad.

✦ **Thyroid malfunction** can also contribute to mild depression, as the thyroid gland slows down after childbirth and may not produce sufficient hormones. The symptoms of a malfunctioning thyroid are lethargy, melancholy, headaches, greater sensitivity to cold, difficulties in speaking, disrupted menstrual periods, and hair loss.

✦ **Anemia**, caused by a decrease in the number of red blood cells, brings about an iron deficiency that will intensify feelings of fatigue and, as a consequence, may lead to mild depression. This problem can be detected easily with a blood test and is cured by iron supplements and a diet of iron-rich foods (many new mothers may prefer to take slow-absorbing iron pills whose effect is less constipating). See pages 136 and 137 for nutritional tips.

✦ **A potassium deficiency** can translate into a feeling of lethargy. It is also detectable through a blood test, and can be treated with a potassium-rich diet (bananas, tomatoes, and oranges).

## *Emotional Causes*

These days, we often hear that "pregnancy is not an illness," that giving birth is painless and easy. Possibly in reaction to the normality of pregnancy and childbirth today, some women seek to "upgrade" the event as if it were some sort of "professional promotion" that deserves a reward. It is now common to hear women speak of a "successful" delivery, as though giving birth was equivalent to passing an exam. For example, many new mothers now expect a gift from the baby's father as a reward for the delivery. These women may relish the first few weeks after childbirth when they are surrounded with congratulatory messages and visits from their family and friends. Then, when all the rejoicing grinds to a halt, they find themselves alone all day with a crying baby and a fat body. Suddenly, the glamour and attention of pregnancy and childbirth seems a distant memory, replaced by sleepless nights and dirty diapers. This realization is enough to send more than one new mother into an emotional slump.

Many women feel they are losing control of their life during the weeks after childbirth. During pregnancy, they may have felt that their body was escaping their control. Beyond proper nutrition and a healthy lifestyle, a pregnant woman cannot control the development of the baby inside her. Giving birth is itself a completely involuntary act. Then once the baby is born, his mother will realize rapidly that she is an individual who, though completely dependent, has her own rhythms and needs that may differ considerably from those of her mother. Babies brings a kind of chaos—fortunately, most of us get used to it.

All new mothers remark that they have trouble achieving anything in a day but the most basic household tasks. This may be deeply disturbing to some women, particularly those who have attained senior professional positions and who led highly organized lives before the baby's birth. They may, consciously or subconsciously, refuse to "let go" for a few weeks, to flow with the baby's rhythms. Sometimes they look to escape from this "unproductive" life by returning to work before they have rested properly.

An obsession with perfection, expectations that are set too high, will lead almost inevitably to anger and frustration. This may happen when a new mother is in competition with other women or her own mother and tries to do "even more" to prove that she can be a better mother, or deliberately does the opposite to show her disapproval. Similarly, a woman who seeks a "perfect" loving relationship with her baby is bound to feel disappointed. Unfortunately, many new mothers today simply "try too hard."

A perfectionist, who has read everything and prepared for every detail of the baby's arrival as if motherhood were a science, may then expect every aspect of her baby's life to fit into well-defined boxes. If childbirth, or the baby, then presents the slightest complication, she may feel hurt and betrayed. Her self-esteem may take a real blow. Or she may feel extremely guilty if she cannot satisfy perfectly the baby's needs. Many new mothers worry excessively the first time that their baby is sick. Fortunately, with time, most learn to relax.

## Socioeconomic Causes

✦ Loneliness and the feeling of losing her identity as a woman can have truly debilitating effects on a new mother. Staying home all day with a baby is particularly hard to tolerate for a woman who was very active in her professional life. In some cases, the loneliness is due to the fact that the mother moved to a new house just before giving birth. She may not know her new neighborhood well. Before moving, she probably had a group of friends and now has no such network. Absence of public transportation, a delicate or sick baby, or severe weather conditions are all reasons why a new mother may be housebound against her will.

✦ Financial and professional insecurity is the source of real worries, especially if the new mother has any doubts about whether she will be able to return to her job or if she fears the reactions of her boss or colleagues. If the baby's father is faced with unemployment, or if their couple's financial situation was not strong before the baby arrived, the mother's concerns may turn to real anguish.

✦ The father's negative reactions towards the baby are another source of real worry. If the father is disturbed by the baby's arrival, especially if he feels jealous or frustrated, a mother's sense of insecurity will increase. She wants to make her husband happy and keep the couple intact (often, subconsciously, in order to ensure her child's financial and emotional security), but she is disturbed by the father's indifference or even hostility to the child. Instead of feeling supported and loved, she may feel downtrodden and often depressed.

## The Solutions

It is essential to call for help before sinking into a real postnatal depression. All the means available should be tried to overcome feelings of anxiety and melancholy. Sometimes, all it takes to get through a rough period is a more regular routine of naps and short recreational breaks, a few alternative treatments, and relaxation skills. But, if symptoms begin to look more like depression (see the tables on pages 230 to 232), then a specialist must be consulted.

## A FEW ORGANIZATIONAL TIPS

- Never go out two evenings in a row.
- Delegate, delegate, delegate, and forget about what you cannot delegate.
- Give your partner a list of daily responsibilities for the baby's care and then leave him to do them at his speed and in the way he wishes to. Babies have an amazing capacity to adapt—and to express dissatisfaction. It is better to leave the room than to stand criticizing behind your partner.
- Avoid saying to the baby's father: "You never help me." Instead, encourage him to think about how happy he makes you when he helps you.
- At the beginning of every day, chart out a simple program (just enough to give the day some structure) that includes at least one or two hours for yourself, as well as an hour or two in the company of another adult.
- Don't assign yourself more than two tasks each day beyond those required in looking after the baby.
- Keep at least one room in your home tidy and looking nice. You can go there when your spirits need a lift.
- Face each problem one step at a time. Your self-esteem will grow with each small solution.

## Coping with Insomnia

Insomnia is a sign of depression. Try the following if you are having trouble sleeping:

- Avoid caffeine and all other stimulants.
- Do some stretching or exercises in the morning or early afternoon.
- Eat dinner early, but avoid going to bed hungry.
- Don't use your bed as a library or a desk; your bed should be associated with sleep.
- Only go to bed when you are tired.
- If you don't fall asleep after ten or fifteen minutes, go to another room and do something boring.
- Make your goal relaxing rather than sleeping.
- Drink a cup of hot milk, or eat a starch (bread, cereal, and pasta) before bed.
- Get up at the same time every day.

+ Turn your alarm clock toward the wall so you cannot see the time.
+ Try drinking an infusion of hops and skullcap before bed.

## Rest

About six weeks after childbirth, you can begin reestablishing a more regular schedule. It is important to let the baby sleep as much as possible in his crib, avoiding short naps in the car or while on a walk. These lead to naps at home that are too short for you to get anything accomplished (including napping yourself). Try to teach the baby to sleep alone during the day by letting him cry a little bit in his cradle. He will sleep better at night, and will start sleeping through the night sooner, if he has become accustomed to this. Don't despair, with time every baby will learn to go to sleep by himself.

If you become really tired, find some help for the "night shift," or even on every other night or for a few hours every afternoon, so that you can get some uninterrupted sleep. Unplug the telephone. Avoid doing housework or errands during these precious nap times.

Many women go through a slump between the eighth and tenth week after childbirth when the accumulated lack of sleep really begins to cause damage. This is the time when depressive thoughts may begin to surface.

## Recreation

For once, having fun is just as important as working!

+ Schedule one fun activity each day: go out with the baby to run errands, see a friend, take a walk. Better yet, go out without the baby.
+ Plan ahead at least three occasions per month when you can go out alone with your partner or a friend.
+ Try to organize activities with friends who also have young babies so that you can take turns baby-sitting. For instance, go to the pool together: one mother can watch the babies while the other swims a few laps, then switch. Or go shopping together: one can watch the babies while the other one tries on clothes.

### Contact with the outside world

+ Try to read the newspaper or watch the news every day.
+ Invite friends to your home who will talk about topics other than the baby.
+ Try to involve your partner with other couples that have young babies: this will help him see that you are not the only mother who is completely swamped.
+ "Mommy and me" groups or other gatherings of young mothers with or without a specialist (nurse, midwife, therapist) in attendance now exist in almost every town. They may be organized by local churches and synagogues, community groups, local libraries, nursing mothers' groups, or the La Leche League. They provide an opportunity for exchanging information with other mothers, getting questions answered by a specialist, doing a few stretches or learning baby massage, and just getting out of the house.

### Diet

Keeping blood sugar levels stable is important to your brain because it is highly dependent on blood sugar as a fuel. Mothers who skip meals or go for long periods without food find themselves becoming irritable and fatigued.

Certain vitamins and nutrients also play an important role in controlling emotions:

+ **Lecithin** helps to build certain neurotransmitters that regulate moods and feelings. New mothers need 200 milligrams per day of this nutrient, which can be found in fish, liver, cauliflower, cabbage, green beans, rice, soy, peanuts, split peas, and wheat germ.
+ **Vitamin B$_5$** (Pantothenic Acid) is also known as the "anti-stress" vitamin and is a major source of energy for the adrenal glands. It is easily depleted by antibiotics. A new mother requires 25 to 50 milligrams per day of this vitamin, which can be found in eggs, fish, poultry, blue cheese, whole grains, lentils, corn, peas, avocados, cauliflower, sweet potatoes, green beans, peanuts, and sunflower seeds.

## MILD DEPRESSION

### Herbal Remedies
### Aromatherapy

Essential oil of Neroli is recommended to ease nervous tensions and anxiety and Chamomile for general soothing and calming. Rose is especially useful for baby blues. Jasmine is another good antidepressant, especially when inhaled or massaged into the skin.

### Homeopathy

- If you are feeling morose, negative, and fearful: take Cimifuga 5C three times a day.
- If you are feeling emotional, excited, very influencible: take Pulsatilla 5C three times a day.
- If you are feeling overwhelmed, underappreciated: take Sepia 5C three times a day.
- If you are feeling sad, disappointed: take Ignatia 5C three times a day.
- If you have imaginary fears about your health: take Phosphorous 5C three times a day.
- If you have settled into a pattern of grief or disappointment and it is becoming the source of physical complaints: take Natrum Muriaticum 5C three times a day.

+ **Vitamin E** regulates neurotransmissions between the brain cells—and plays a role in controlling headaches. A new mother should absorb 8 to 12 milligrams per day of this vitamin, which can be found in wheat germ oil, whole wheat flour, seeds, almonds, dried beans, corn oil, peanut oil, safflower oil, and green leafy vegetables.

+ **Zinc** is extremely important to all metabolic functions. Many depressive mothers have been found to be zinc-deficient. The average daily intake recommended for new mothers is 12 to 30 milligrams per day.

# Managing Stress

Stress can best be defined as the way in which an organism reacts to its environment. Stress can be sudden in the case of major events, or chronic as a result of repeated aggression. For humans, stress occurs when living conditions change, during difficult life passages, when major adaptation is required due to societal or professional constraints, or in a difficult environment. Contrary to popular belief, stress is not caused by a "stressful situation" but by a person's coping mechanism and reactions to the situation. Therefore, stress can produce feelings of satisfaction, happiness, even euphoria when a person is able to cope with the situation, or it may lead to illness, fatigue, or even a breakdown when a person is unable to cope adequately.

Giving birth is a particularly intense event, as is divorce, the death or serious illness of a close relative, marriage, or loss of a job. The reactions of the body and the mind to childbirth are proportional to the upheaval in your life caused by the baby's arrival. A career woman who manages a demanding work schedule nevertheless may find great difficulty in coping with her demanding infant.

It is equally interesting to note that, during pregnancy and the postnatal period, a woman's dreams are more vivid, more colorful, more elaborate, and sometimes more troubling. A woman who is pregnant or has just given birth is also more likely to remember her dreams. This is due to the excitement, stress, and subconscious internal conflicts that surface during her sleep. Hormonal changes often cause more intense dreams, which tend to be a more memorable dreams. A new mother also wakes more often during the night, which makes it easier for her to remember her dreams. Also, it has been proven that we remember our dreams better during periods of change or stress.

If the new mother's sleep is disturbed, her reactions during waking hours may be more hostile or aggressive than normal, because she is in

*Ancient prayer: "God give me the strength to change what I can, the courage to accept what I cannot change, and the wisdom to know the difference."*

fact more vulnerable. The simplest problem may "ruin her day" or even seem insurmountable.

Physical signs of stress include a rapid heartbeat and faster breathing, increased adrenaline flow, muscle tension, fatigue, loss of concentration, and a weakened immune system that is more susceptible to infection. Psychological stress impairs the efficiency of the immune system. Studies have shown that 42 percent of new mothers experience a notable increase in the respiratory illnesses in their first year. However, if stress can be channeled, it can be transformed into a positive source of energy.

## Stressful Situations

Coping with stress depends entirely on how you view the stressful situation. Does it seem insurmountable or a stimulating challenge? The difference between these two responses to the same situation comes from a person's nature: some people thrive in stressful situations, others lose their grip.

The important thing is not to react as a passive victim, but to know how to evaluate the situation, recognizing when stress is becoming damaging, and then to respond in order to reduce the potential adverse effects of stress. This technique is fundamental for a new mother, who is often confronted with choices: "The baby is finally sleeping—should I use this time to cook a nice dinner for my partner (who has been complaining that he hasn't eaten well since the baby arrived) or should I take the nap I really need?" Knowing how to take things in hand and control your daily life can greatly help you overcome these challenges.

Unfortunately, the "stressful situation" can be a mother or a mother-in-law, a dear friend, or another person who may feel hurt because you cannot see them so often just now. But don't forget that during the postnatal period, your priorities are your baby and yourself. During these few weeks, it is much more important to eliminate potentially stressful situations than to try to please other people.

## Relaxation

Managing stress requires some "time out" and an evaluation of the situation, as well as inner calm and a reserve of energy.

Relaxing is especially important before nursing. For many new mothers who find it hard to go back to sleep after a feeding session in the middle of the night, relaxation can also be useful. When all our worries (and our growing "to do" list) prevent us from taking a nap even when the baby is sleeping, a short relaxation session can be just as beneficial as an hour of fitful sleep. A relaxed mother will be more optimistic and less anxious.

When a person is relaxed, her pulse rate, her brainwaves, and her breathing will all slow down: just the opposite of the classic reaction to stress. Yoga, meditation, and gentle stretches can help you to reach this state. A sense of peace and relaxation is often also felt following a bout of strenuous exercise because exercise releases the endorphins and encephalins of the body, which are its natural antidepressants. Whether it be biking, walking, aerobics, or kickboxing, it's important to choose an activity that appeals to you. Rather than describing each of these techniques in detail, we advise you to try a few classes or, if you have no such resources in your area, a book or a video.

### An Exercise for Stress Relief

+ Sit on a chair or armchair that supports you well, with your feet placed flat on a low stool or on a book (so that your thigh muscles are relaxed).
+ Let your legs open naturally from the hip, wiggle your toes to release any tension. Place your hands comfortably on your thighs, the fingers slightly separated. Close your eyes.
+ Be aware of your body, the places where it is touching the chair and the floor. Exhale, and let go.
+ Concentrate on your breathing, and imagine that each time you exhale, some of the tension is flowing out of your body.
+ Think about relaxing your shoulders, letting them fall. Stretch your neck. Let go of your stomach muscles.
+ Wiggle your fingers and toes again. Stretch. Yawn, and open your eyes.

It is important not to do this exercise for too long, especially in the beginning, because it is difficult to concentrate for long periods of time. You do not want the relaxation session to turn into another "worry session."

Since a new mother probably has only about five minutes at a time to spend doing relaxation exercises, she should learn to be aware of her body throughout the day. For example, try sticking a Post-it note over the baby's changing table. Every time you change the baby, become aware of the tension in your back and shoulders. The more you are aware of the tension in your body, the more you can control it.

## Relaxing positions

After a physical effort or a tense situation, take a few minutes to get into one of these positions so as to "recover."

Sitting at a table, put your head down onto your arms, folded in a "cradle."

Lie on the floor on your stomach, with a pillow under your hips and another beneath your head. This is an excellent position for comforting hemorrhoid or perineum pain in the days following childbirth.

Lying on your back, again with pillows under your hips and head, open your legs slightly and turn your palms toward the ceiling.

Lie on your back with a pillow beneath your head, and raise your legs onto a low table, foot stool, or large pillow.

Sit in a squatting position on your heels (if this isn't too painful), your chest resting on two sofa cushions piled one on the other, with your arms over your head, also resting on the cushions. This position is also a good back stretch.

## Breathing

This is one of the most efficient ways to reach a relaxed state, because breathing is the first body function affected by stress. Whenever you find yourself confronting a difficult situation (there are no diapers left and it's eight o'clock on Saturday night; the baby has just vomited all over his clean sheets at three A.M.), exhale a long, slow breath. Wait a moment. Then inhale.

## Postnatal Depression

| | How many women are affected? | When does it start? | How long does it last? | What can be done? |
|---|---|---|---|---|
| **Mild Depressive State** | Almost all new mothers | Anytime in the first four months—usually worst 8 weeks after childbirth when sleep deprivation is at its height | Usually disappears around 12 weeks when the baby's sleep patterns are more established (unless there is a serious health problem or with twins) | • Help, rest<br>• Support networks<br>• Alternative remedies<br>• Diet<br>• Solving any physical problems<br>• Relaxation |
| **Postnatal Depression** | 1 woman in 10 | Anytime in the first year. About 50 percent of postnatal depressions begin about 2 weeks after childbirth; 15 percent occur within 2 to 6 weeks; and the rest begin at least 3 months postpartum. | If left untreated, can last for years | Specialized treatment, including medication, psychotherapy, and alternative complementary remedies |
| **Puerperal Psychosis** | 1 mother in 1,000 | 50 percent occur immediately after childbirth, the remaining within the first 2 weeks | Usually lasts about 11 weeks; if left untreated, can last for years | Hospitalization; psychiatric treatment |

### Mild Depressive State

Bouts of depression occur periodically

Tired, but feels better after a few good nights

### Postnatal Depression

Continually depressed

Perpetually tired. Rest and sleep do not bring relief. Insomnia at night but desires to nap throughout the day. Nightmares. Mental tiredness: no energy, no interest in things.

## Mild Depressive State

Tears flow at the slightest setback or frustration

Often absentminded, forgetful

Neglects domestic tasks. The home, other children feel like a huge burden. Demoralized but tries to cope.

Feels isolated from the outside world

Irritable

Extremely sensitive, reacts strongly to bad news

Questions her ability to be a good mother. Feels guilty. Lacks self-confidence.

## Postnatal Depression

Cries without reason, or else incapable of crying despite strong urge to do so

Forgets even important things (taking care of the baby), then feels extremely guilty to the point of not daring to leave the house. Great difficulty in concentration.

Feels overwhelmed. Distress affects all her reactions. Total lack of self-esteem. Feels paralyzed.

Feels unwanted, criticized. Jealous of other mothers who seem to cope better. Feels cut off from the rest of the world as if by a glass wall.

Fits of anger (especially with women who appeared to have a lot of self-control). Self-destructive. May be abusive with the baby (but hides this by appearing excessively affectionate in public).

Anxiety attacks. Lack of interest for the outside world. Feels numb toward the baby.

Excessive or irrational guilt about the birth, her success at breast-feeding, or the baby's appearance. Thinks that the baby was mistake. Feels incompetent. Feels that she is being constantly criticized.

## Mild Depressive State

Neglects her appearance. May focus only on the baby's clothes.

Irregular eating habits

Little interest in sex

Physical symptoms linked to fatigue: backache, stomach ache, headache

## Postnatal Depression

Convinced that something terrible is going to happen, that her baby or partner is in danger. In the worst case: suicidal tendencies.

Obsessive about food or complete indifference toward food

Complete absence of libido

Physical symptoms such as palpitations, difficulty in breathing, hair loss in large amounts, cramps. Hypochondria.

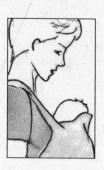

# 19

# Postnatal Depression

This illness is often misdiagnosed because our culture continues to believe firmly in the myth of "maternal bliss." The image of a joyful, relaxed mother holding a contented newborn while the smiling father looks on proudly is the one which comes to mind for most of us when we hear the sentence "she's just had a baby." And it's still the icon used by media, advertising, and even religious institutions to convey the concept of motherhood. If the baby appears healthy and thriving, we simply take it for granted that his mother is happy and well. So when things are not so rosy, when the mother is distraught or apathetic, we don't quite know how to react. Rather than encourage her to seek professional help, we tend to turn our backs in shame and embarrassment, or pretend that a problem does not exist.

The person closest to the mother who can witness the symptoms of postnatal or postpartum depression first is naturally her partner. He is the one who should convince her to see specialists and organize her care. However, this is not a topic that men discuss among themselves nor hear about in the media. So the father may be even more disoriented and worried about what is happening to his spouse. Family and friends therefore can play a vital role in helping him cope with the situation.

Most of us know that postnatal depression exists, but few of us are capable of recognizing its symptoms. Several of these symptoms (such as great excitability) are not typical of the gloom and despondency we normally associate with depression. The chart on pages 230–232 may be useful in distinguishing between "baby blues," fatigue-induced depression, and the psychiatric illness that medical textbooks refer to as postnatal depression.

## Symptoms of Postnatal Depression

Here is a quick rundown:

+ A high level of excitability that is characterized by the inability to sleep, frenetic activity that can lead to collapse, irritability, confused language, and difficulty in concentrating or reasoning properly. This state usually starts shortly after childbirth and can therefore be confused with the euphoria many mothers feel in the first days after a baby's birth.

+ A feeling of panic that is manifested by extreme anxiety, inexplicable panic attacks, physical reactions such as palpitations, hot flashes, trembling, dizziness, excessive sweating, numbness, and tingling in the hands and feet, or even an impression of suffocation. Panic attacks are sometimes brought on by a situation that reminds the new mother of a past trauma.

+ Obsessive thoughts and fantasies. Unlike the woman suffering from puerperal psychosis (see page 242), who "hears voices" commanding her to harm herself or the baby, a depressed woman knows that she is fantasizing and can control herself. But she may feel extremely guilty about such thoughts and can sometimes undertake complicated rituals to protect herself.

### Predispositions to Postnatal Depression

Postnatal depression can strike any healthy woman, regardless of the number of children she has, her socioeconomic level, her religion, ethnic group, cultural origins, or whether or not she is breast-feeding.

However, certain women are at greater risk if they present the following characteristics:

+ Previous psychological troubles.
+ Postnatal depression after a previous childbirth.
+ Heredity (mother, aunt, or sister have had this problem). In addition to a genetic predisposition, women who have seen their own mothers suffer from depression are more prone to depression themselves.
+ A bad experience during fertility treatments.
+ A difficult pregnancy.

If a future mother thinks that she falls into one of these groups, she is well advised to alert her doctor about her concerns before she gives birth. With the proper professional support, which may include medication, a woman with high-risk factors today can greatly reduce her probability of undergoing a severe depression.

## The Causes of Postnatal Depression

### Biochemical Causes

As has been described elsewhere in this book, the body's progesterone and estrogen levels increase gradually over the nine months of pregnancy reach levels some thirty to fifty times higher than normal. Then, in less than three days after the baby's birth, these levels drop dramatically. Since estrogen and progesterone have an antidepressive effect on the brain, such a violent shift will almost inevitably affect our emotions. After childbirth, the surge of prolactin (the hormone that allows milk production) also hinders the production of progesterone and estrogen. Even if a woman does not breast-feed, her prolactin levels are sufficiently high to have an influence on estrogen and progesterone for almost two months.

As we mentioned at the beginning of this section, each woman will react differently to the hormonal turmoil occurring in her body. Some will adjust rapidly with almost no impact on her mood or state of mind. One woman in ten will succumb to the overwhelming feeling of despair that is genuine postnatal depression.

To make matters more complicated, one cause can hide another.

Hormones can cause physical reactions that trigger the release or cause the obstruction of further hormones. For example, carbohydrates are needed for the body to manufacture progesterone. So if a woman is distraught and loses her appetite, she will not only lack in energy but also deprive her body of the ingredients it needs to produce the hormones that will make her feel better. As we noted on pages 140–141, this is an important reason not to begin dieting too soon after childbirth.

## Emotional Causes

Reactions to childbirth are another cause of postnatal depression. As we discussed in Chapter 18, a mother's emotional response to childbirth is not always one of joy. Some specialists consider that severe, negative reactions can induce psychological tensions that are the major cause of postnatal depression. For example, a woman may be deeply disturbed by the feeling of "losing control" during delivery. Usually, such women are reluctant to accept their powerlessness when faced with such an overwhelming physical transformation. Likewise, a woman who went through her pregnancy in a state of anger and frustration with her body will find to her surprise that these feelings tend to persist after childbirth. She probably will be more tired than will a woman who experienced a more tranquil pregnancy. And fatigue, as we have seen, can rapidly lead to depression.

Depression is not caused by a difficult delivery, but, combined with other factors such as loneliness or material hardship, a bad birth experience can lead to psychological difficulties.

The mother's psychological past is yet another cause of depression. Unresolved grief (such as after a divorce, or following the loss of a parent or loved one) or psychological traumas dating from the mother's childhood or adolescence (sexual or physical abuse, abandonment)—all these issues may resurface or suddenly appear overwhelming to the mother immediately after childbirth, threatening her self-confidence and her ability to bond with her new baby.

## External Factors

Stressful relationships also contribute to postnatal depression. Before her pregnancy, a woman may have handled tension reasonably well within her relationships with her partner or with her parents and in-laws. Once the baby is born, her impulse is to protect her from stressful situations by acting as a kind of "emotional shield." Given the heightened psychological vulnerability of any new mother, this sort of pressure can rapidly bring her to the edge of depression. In serious situations, such as when the father is violent or has a problem with substance abuse, outside help is essential as the mother simply will not be able to cope alone.

Social isolation also contributes to the problem. According to the British midwife Sheila Kitzinger, social isolation, together with poverty, is one of the primary causes of depression among women with young children. If a woman finds herself alone with her baby for more than eight hours a day, if she is housebound due to lack of transportation or severe weather conditions, if she has no extended family to give support, she will have no one with whom to share her feelings, no one to help in practical ways. Every woman needs contact with other "grown-ups" to reaffirm her identity as an autonomous adult, not just as a mother. As stated by Kitzinger: "Being depressed because she is isolated has nothing to do with a woman's early infantile experience, her relationship with her mother, her emotional immaturity, or her hormones. She is depressed because the environment makes mothering an almost impossible task." Some psychologists have found that women who return to work after childbirth are less susceptible to postnatal depression than women who stay home alone. (Tips on how to break out of isolation can be found on pages 223–224).

A difficult baby, a baby who cries constantly, sleeps little, who seems hypersensitive and sullen, or who has health complications such as colic or reflux, is extremely tiring. Faced with this small creature that they cannot seem to soothe, the parents may feel both frustrated and guilty.

## Consequences for the Family

Postnatal depression almost inevitably causes tension within a relationship. The woman may feel abandoned; her partner may feel like a victim. Although it is a difficult time for both, small gestures by the father, such as accompanying his wife to her therapy sessions, can create a lot of goodwill.

Women suffering from depression usually worry about the effect of their illness on the baby. They need to be reassured that there is no time limit for establishing a strong mother-child bond, no critical point after which all is lost. Once the situation has been resolved, a mother can "make up for lost time." Her priority is to seek treatment fast—not to hope that the depression will just "go away with time"—so that her illness will be cured before its effects leave a permanent mark on the family.

Nevertheless, it is important to explain to any older children that their mother is not well, that she will get better, that it is not their fault, nor is it the fault of the baby. But one cannot expect the older children to take over family duties and responsibilities beyond their abilities.

## Healing the Mind

In the case of a true postnatal depression, nonmedical remedies are not sufficient. Those who say that "all you need is a little will power" are causing a great disservice to all women. Postnatal depression is an illness that can only be cured with specialized help.

### When to Call on Specialists

According to Drs. Anne Dunnewold and Diane Sanford, a mother should seek specialized help when:

+ If at six weeks after childbirth the situation seems to be getting worse: she is still just as tired, depressed and overwhelmed.
+ Her symptoms are strong enough to disrupt her daily activities/routine.
+ The nonmedical treatments and suggestions mentioned on pages 221 to 225 have been tried for at least ten days and seem to have no effect.
+ A person she respects advises her to consult a doctor.
+ She can no longer manage to care for the baby or herself.
+ She is afraid that she will harm the baby or herself.
+ She has no appetite or, on the contrary, is bingeing on food (in other words, exhibiting signs of anorexia or bulimia).

### Difficulties in Diagnosis

Ideally, all women at risk for postnatal depression would be identified during their pregnancies so that preventive treatment could begin immediately after delivery. In reality, its early diagnosis is hindered by a number of obstacles: if a mother's postnatal checkup six weeks after the baby's birth is a little too rushed, the doctor may miss the symptoms of postnatal depression. Furthermore, in 40 percent of cases, depression sets in *after* the routine postnatal visit that is often a mother's last contact with the medical world. She may consult her primary caregiver or internist, complaining of fatigue, insomnia, and especially backaches (depression can be masked by physical symptoms that are actually only a transference of emotional suffering). She may even transpose her own ailments onto her child, and be continually rushing to the pediatrician. But if her physician or the pediatrician is not trained to detect postnatal depression, they may simply prescribe vitamins or physical therapy and not refer the mother to an appropriate specialist. The most pernicious aspect of postnatal depression is the way it can be hidden behind symptoms that distract doctors and lead them farther away from the real cause. Indeed, the treatment of postnatal depression requires a complex knowledge of several disciplines: psychiatry, obstetrics, endocrinology, as well as general medicine.

An appropriate treatment will require a combination of prescription drugs and psychotherapy, and, if the woman so desires, a number of alternative treatments that can lessen the side effects of psychiatric medication (homeopathy, aromatherapy, acupuncture, osteopathy, and relaxation techniques).

**The first step toward recovery is taking action. If a doctor seems not to take your situation seriously and tells you that you are only going through a rough patch on the road, see another doctor.**

## Psychiatric Medication

It is crucial to understand that prescription drugs will only halt the downward spiral. They will allow a woman to feel more self-confidence and self-esteem. But medication will not treat the cause of the problem. For this reason, psychotherapy is an essential component of the treatment for postnatal depression.

## Which Medication?

Medical research in antidepressant medication is progressing constantly. This category of prescription drugs already has gone through three "generations" of improvements. Today, SSRIs (selective serotonin reuptake inhibitors) are the most often prescribed (one of the most commonly prescribed drugs is Prozac). They act by restoring the correct chemical processes in the brain. Their effect is slow (it can take up to four weeks to begin to see results), but conclusive.

Used alone or in combination with antidepressants, tranquilizers have the advantage of immediate effectiveness. They can help overcome moments of anguish, and help the body relax. However, they can in some cases cause the opposite effect by increasing rather than diminishing the feelings of unease. Some are quite sedative while others do not cause drowsiness. (*Warning*: Breast-feeding is contraindicated if undergoing this treatment.)

Tranquilizers can cause dependency and should not be prescribed for longer than three months. They work by suppressing the symptoms of depression, especially anguish, but they do not cure them. Again, psychotherapy is an essential part of the cure.

## For How Long?

The length of treatment varies from one individual to another, but usually medication must be maintained for four to six months *after* the symptoms disappear. Several different drugs or combinations of drugs may need to be tried before the right treatment is found. If no improvement is noticed after three or four weeks of a certain medication, it's time to change treatment.

## What About Breast-feeding?

This is a sensitive topic. For some depressed mothers, nursing is one of the few ways they can express their maternal love and provide for the baby's needs. It is one of their only sources of self-esteem. An abrupt decision to wean the baby will cause a second hormonal drop, and even stronger emotional repercussions. However, the long-term effects of antidepressants are not known. Therefore, most doctors recommend that the mother stop breast-feeding or else use an earlier "generation" of prescription drugs whose side effects are better known and whose long-term effects on the baby who absorbs them through breast milk

## A FEW HINTS

- Avoid therapists who seem to underestimate the importance of the postpartum period in a woman's life.
- It is perfectly normal to meet several therapists before settling on one. It is impossible to open up to a person with whom you don't get along or who doesn't seem to understand you. Follow your intuition; the stakes are high. There are enough therapists around for you to change if you have the slightest doubt.
- Never forget that you are "in the driver's seat." Never allow the therapist to make you feel badly or to treat you with condescension.

have been studied. The decision is not an easy one. Pros and cons must be weighed carefully, taking into consideration the baby's age and the length of time she has been breast-fed.

## Psychotherapy

There is no set protocol for treatment of postpartum depression, but psychotherapy can be an integral part of any plan, whether it includes drug therapy or not.

### How to Choose a Therapist

This is one specialist you should not select from the phone book. Ideally, a doctor will recommend someone he or she knows based on his or her reputation within the medical community. Because it is essential for a woman to trust her therapist, it is very important that she be reassured at the outset by outward signs of credibility, such as the appropriate diplomas and accreditation that document training in psychiatry, psychoanalysis, or clinical psychology.

### Complementary Treatments

In combination with the medical and psychological treatments described above, alternative treatments can speed the healing process and minimize any negative side effects from the prescription medication. These include homeopathy, aromatherapy, acupuncture, osteopathy, nutrition therapy, and various relaxation techniques. Again, it is important to consult reputable, accredited practitioners (see above on how to choose a practitioner), often a medical doctor who has further specialized in alternative therapies. Beware of practitioners who attempt to convince you to stop your prescription medication or give you advice contrary to that of your psychiatrist. In most cases of postnatal depression, alternative treatments should be seen as complementary and not as a substitute for medical treatments.

## Puerperal Psychosis

This extremely serious psychiatric illness affects about one woman in a thousand. The illness surfaces in the two weeks following childbirth, and lasts about eleven weeks. During this period, a woman undergoes an emotional upheaval so severe that she can no longer sleep. She may suffer from memory loss, complete confusion, or hallucinations—as if she were living in a dream. She may hear voices telling her to harm the baby. She usually appears extremely agitated, obsessive (for example, continually washing her hands or cleaning the house), or paralyzed by fear, yet she will not realize that she is delirious.

As this illness usually occurs soon after childbirth and has such severe symptoms, it is often detected even before a mother leaves the hospital. It requires immediate admittance to a psychiatric hospital (there are more and more hospitals with psychiatric units especially designed for young mothers and their babies). If treated in time, most women recover completely with a combination of antidepressants, tranquilizers, and antidelirium drugs, followed by a course of psychotherapy.

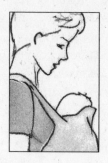

# 20

# The Mother in You

Becoming a mother does not mean losing our identity as a wife or partner in a couple, as a professional, and above all, as a unique individual. But many new mothers will find themselves wondering how one person can handle all these roles.

## Maternal Instinct—Is It in All of Us?

For years, the notion of a "maternal instinct" was used to justify assigning to women all the tasks associated with raising children. Today, feminists oppose this argument and the debate has intensified over the past few decades. Are all women really meant by nature to be the caregivers? Some psychologists dispute the existence of an "instinct" that is found in some humans (women) and not in others (men). Some writers offer a more mechanical explanation for the relationship that develops between a mother and her child: in order to satisfy his needs, the child prompts his mother by crying or smiling, for example, and the mother is genetically programmed to respond to these signals. Others describe the instinctive need a mother feels to transmit to her child

those psychological capacities that differentiate humans from animals—for example, a sensitivity to others, a perception of the world, or
an awareness of one's own body.

Where do all of these theories leave us? Undeniably, new feelings
awaken in us during pregnancy under the influence of hormonal
secretions from the placenta. These sensations are reinforced with the
release of the prolactin hormone when we breast-feed or cuddle our
baby. Somehow, over time, we seem to have an intuitive understanding of the baby. Whether we call this sensation "instinct" or something else, it has ensured the survival of newborn humans since time
began. Today, however, these natural feelings are often stifled in a
society that frowns upon spontaneous expressions of maternal
instinct: sleeping with our baby, nursing on demand, carrying the
baby around with us. This may explain why some mothers experience motherhood as a burden, and wait impatiently for the time
when their child will finally be independent. In the meantime, they
call on as many outside caregivers as possible to minimize their own
involvement.

The maternal instinct, if it exists, functions primarily at the subconscious level. Therefore, we mothers need something a little more conscious and concrete to give us the strength, energy, and joy we need to
take good care of our babies day in and day out. It is maternal love that
makes us want to spend the time it takes to understand our child, to
teach him gently that he is not all-powerful, so that one day he can fly
on his own wings.

However, learning to love a child takes time. It requires far more
commitment than is advertised by a society that would often have us
think that women are turned into mothers simply through the biological act of giving birth and the impact of a few hormones.

## The "Perfect Mother"

In the eighteenth century, one in three children died before their first
birthday, and only half of all children could expect to live to the age of
twenty-one. Mothers didn't love their children less, but their emotional
investment probably differed from ours. When infant mortality rates
dropped at the beginning of the nineteenth century, it was no longer
necessary to produce as many children to ensure a family's survival. As

a result, couples began attempting to control their family size. While in 1860, there was an average of 6 children per family, this statistic had plummeted to 2.3 children by 1924. For the first time, the notion of choice entered into the reproductive process.

Inevitably, this new dimension had a major impact on parental emotions that continue to this day: fewer children per family means a greater emotional investment in each child. It also means more worries about each one. Parents have more difficulty in being separated from their children; they feel guilty when they become irritated or angry with them. Today, we are almost obsessed with our children's development: their first tooth, their first step, and their intellectual abilities. We never tire of discussing these issues with other mothers (and comparing our child to theirs). We seem to find any excuse to justify spending money on their clothes and toys. And the environment in which we are raising our children also preoccupies us—politicians certainly understand how to pull on our heartstrings when they refer to the "world our children will live in" in their speeches! Many young mothers find that they can no longer stand to watch the news or television programs containing violence or misery.

The myth of the "happy mother" has long been perpetuated by our religious institutions, by our governments, even by our own mothers. But the world in which they were born is almost unrecognizable today. When our grandmothers and mothers gave birth, they generally benefited from a strong support network of family and other sources of help, due in large part to the fact that they stayed in bed much longer. Fewer women worked outside the home and women probably had fewer professional aspirations. Most importantly, they were less well informed (psychology is a recent science), asked fewer questions about their children's emotional development, and usually worried much less than we do about the way in which they were bringing up their children. In contrast, mothers today are more concerned, tenser, and much more sensitive to criticisms from a society that seems to tolerate only "perfect" mothers. Just look at the number of books and magazines we all read on the subject of motherhood! We want yardsticks to evaluate our children's development, yet we worry when they have not achieved the exact level of their peer groups. We are both critical of the way in which we were brought up, but also afraid of what our children might reproach us for in later years.

## THE "GOOD-ENOUGH" MOTHER

- As parents, our obligation is not to raise a perfect child, but to listen and to make ourselves available.
- Parents have less impact on their child's development than the media and many specialists would have us believe. A child's emotional development depends heavily on his own life experiences. Only extreme actions by parents can truly damage their development.
- Every child is an individual. We should accept that he has his own feelings about the world around him and we should be sensitive to these feelings.
- Our child's behavior is not necessarily a reflection of our aptitude as a parent. Babies are born with different temperaments, and therefore will react differently to similar situations.
- Parents have less influence on their child's personality than we may think. A little baby is very forgiving of his mother.

  **The important thing is not what you do; it's how you do it. Follow your intuition. There are no "must-do's" and "mustn't-do's."**

- Don't get caught up in the popular notion of the "perfect start." Regardless of what sort of birth experience you had, the important thing is how your baby's childhood unfolds.
- Don't forget your own needs and those of your relationship.

## As a result . . .

- ✦ This tension may rub off onto our children.
- ✦ Our fears and worries turn into physical problems: fatigue, backaches, and other symptoms of stress.
- ✦ We become overdependent on the advice of specialists. Mothers have never consulted pediatricians as frequently as they do now. When we seek too many outside opinions, our common sense and natural instincts get forgotten.
- ✦ We tend to subordinate all of our needs to those of the baby; the first to suffer are usually our sex life and our relationship with our spouse.
- ✦ We neglect our appearance, thinking that everyone will forgive us because we are, first and foremost, "good mothers."

Well-known British pediatrician and psychologist Donald Winnicott, whose theories are quite comforting to the modern mother, has written about this period in a mother's life. According to him, all women experience a sort of "motherhood crisis," which he terms "normal madness." This state of constant worry and hypersensitivity actually is beneficial and necessary to establish the mother-infant bond, which he calls the "primary maternal preoccupation." He also talks about the "mercilessness" of babies who can't wait, who demand, and who literally "force" us to love them. Dr. Winnicott offers an alternative to the "perfect mother"—the "good enough mother."

Likewise, the feelings of frustration that most mothers experience at some point can also be viewed as nature's way of convincing us to change the way we do things, to try new approaches with our children. It is perfectly normal to find yourself wondering from time to time why you ever had this baby. Any mother "working" twenty-four-hour shifts is bound to feel cranky and bitter. A mother might resent her child for keeping her away from her spouse, especially if at this stage he is acting more like the baby's rival than its father. Mothers who claim never to get mad at their babies probably have a more insidious way of expressing their feelings. It is important that children learn that their parents can be angry with them yet not stop loving them.

A mother cannot be "in love" with her baby all of the time. She sometimes desperately needs to put some distance between herself and that obstinate, selfish little bundle. A baby's demands and needs are limitless. Part of our role as mothers is to place limits on these requests in order to prepare our children for life in society.

Despite all of this, there is undeniably some form of magic involved. How else can you explain that giving so much of yourself is not a chore, but a real pleasure?

However, one fundamental condition is necessary before the "magic" of maternal love can transcend the worry and fatigue of motherhood: a new mother must have resolved any childhood conflicts of her own, and established sufficient distance from her own mother. Many psychologists are quite categorical on this matter: the success of motherhood depends above all on the mother having her own sense of self-esteem.

# The Impact of Our Families

In many countries, childbirth and motherhood are collective acts. Women return to their family home to give birth, children grow up within a joint-family community, and maternal duties are shared by a group of women. Sometimes these women may be in conflict with tyrannical mothers-in-law, but they live in a sort of "sorority" through which they give each other moral support. In Western societies, on the other hand, childbirth and motherhood have become solitary acts. We are often left alone to confront repressed feelings about our childhood and the tensions in our relationship with our parents. These feelings can surface abruptly during the postnatal period.

## Burying Negative Aspects of Our Childhood

It is said that childbirth makes every woman relive her own childhood: the bad memories as well as the good ones. At the birth of their own child, many women are transported back into their memories of their earliest relations with their own mothers, and to the images of motherhood that have been etched in their minds. Without our being aware of it, these images shape the way we become mothers. But this unconscious commemoration does not only bring pain, it actually gives us the tools to identify with our newborn baby, to seek to understand her and to protect her. Secondly, the act of reviving even painful memories, allows a woman to reconcile herself with her childhood, and then to take a crucial step toward becoming a mother herself: to leave her own childhood behind.

This task of resigning yourself to the loss of your own childhood can be undertaken at the onset of pregnancy, after childbirth, or even much later. It consists of accepting the fact that you no longer are your mother's child but that you have become a mother yourself. This is often neither quick nor easy. We may fear that we will "disappear" in the process of ceasing to be a child in order to become a parent, especially if we are afraid of not being able to handle our new responsibilities as a mother. There is also the fear of making our own mothers "disappear" by turning them into grandmothers. This is why some women have such a strong need to be "mothered" while they are going through labor, yet refuse any assistance. Many women want their own mothers around to benefit from their experience, yet they forget that childbirth has changed tremendously in the past twenty-five years, and that their mothers often don't remember very much in detail anyway.

## The Relationship Between Mothers and Grandmothers

A mother is also a daughter, a granddaughter, a niece, or a sister. Her own extended family inevitably will have an impact on how she relates to her own children. Our behavior as a parent—mother or father—is in great part the result of the parents we ourselves had. Whether we want to do as they did, or avoid doing as they did, whether we want to concede to their wishes or oppose them, our parents remain a model by which we steer ourselves.

Others may be afraid of making the same mistakes as their own mothers. As a result, they would rather have someone else raise their children in order to "protect" them. This may appear to be an odd reaction, much frowned upon by society, yet it is founded in love. These women must reconcile themselves with their wounded childhood in order to gain confidence in their abilities as mothers. History repeats itself in all families, but it need not be in a dramatic or negative manner.

In a nutshell, we should neither waste our energy trying to be as perfect as our own mother is, nor should we deliberately attempt to do the opposite so as to prove that our approach is better. This is particularly difficult if your mother or mother-in-law seems to have been the "perfect mother." To this end, you will have to determine how much distance from your parents is necessary for you to establish your own identity as a mother.

### And the Grandparents . . .

Grandparents play an important role in providing our babies with a heritage and a sense of belonging to a family unit. Having a baby makes us conscious of certain patterns of behavior within our extended family, of traditions and customs that we may wish to transmit to our children. We will be relying more heavily on our families now for their emotional, logistical, or financial support. A woman's relationship with her partner's family also changes with the baby's birth as she now has established a blood link; more so than through marriage, she becomes part of the "clan." For these reasons, new mothers will often make a special effort to heal old rifts and tensions within their families.

Nevertheless, it is important to remember that sometimes parents have a hard time becoming grandparents. They are inevitably reminded that time is passing. They may look back on happier days (if they are widowed or ill, for instance), or reflect on the difficulties they had in raising you when you (now a mother yourself) were their child. With the birth of this new baby, your parents step up a notch in the generation ladder, moving closer to death, or at least to the role of "ancestors."

A new grandmother may fear that her daughter does not know how to care for a baby. This explains the healthy doses of advice, frequent phone calls, or unexpected visits that a new mother may experience. The new grandmother may also be a little jealous of her daughter, who now is free to follow her intuition instead of abiding by a set of strict rules. A grandmother who is widowed and alone may find new hope through this baby, and might become a little possessive. Conversely, if the grandmother is dead, lives far away, or is simply too involved in her own life, the new mother and baby may really miss her, as grandparents play an important role in a balanced childhood.

A mother-in-law may worry that her son spends too much time at home now, and that his career will suffer. Sometimes both grandmothers feel insulted if the new mother does not follow their advice to the fullest. It is worse when grandparents are frequently called upon to baby-sit, but are warned not to "interfere" with their grandchildren's upbringing. Just like fathers-to-be, future grandmothers sometimes have accidents or get sick in order to, subconsciously, draw attention to themselves.

Despite all of these potential complications, it is important to begin a dialogue early in your pregnancy so as to share your expectations and establish a few ground rules. One good technique is to show your mother and mother-in-law the baby-care books and articles you are reading, pointing out the issues on which you agree or disagree. This can lead to some very constructive conversations in which you gently, but firmly, establish the boundaries around your future family.

## When Life and Death Become Entangled

A woman whose parent is deceased may suddenly find herself grieving again at the birth of her own child. The feeling of loss will be particularly strong at this time, as she will not have her parent available to

## MOTHER AND DAUGHTER

No matter what the state of your current relationship with your mother, it will change after the birth of your first child.

If you have a difficult relationship with your mother, do not be misled into believing that the baby's arrival will finally bring your mother's approval. You may find it useful to examine these feelings with a therapist.

Once you have your own baby, you may find yourself noticing how much you resemble your mother. Depending on how happy your childhood was, these revelations may be pleasing or irritating.

The baby's arrival is an excellent opportunity to open a dialogue and create a new understanding between a woman and her mother or mother-in-law. This is especially important in the case of religious or racially mixed couples where the baby can provide a link between the two families. A new baby brings faith and hope to all.

recognize her now as a mother, not just as a child. If a woman loses a parent or a loved one while she is pregnant, the mourning process may overwhelm the normally joyous sensation of life growing inside her. At the moment of giving birth, she may find herself submerged in sadness. If this occurs, it is extremely important for the mother to talk to her baby, to tell him that she is not the cause of her mother's grief and that she was not born to replace the dead person.

If an older child has died before the new baby's birth, such dialogue is even more important. Some mothers, who may not have had the opportunity to finish grieving, might unconsciously expect the new baby to replace the previous child. That, clearly, is an impossible task. In both of these cases, trained therapists should be sought to help the mother through this renewed period of mourning.

## Raising a Child

### A Bit of Historical Background

Until the beginning of the twentieth century, a woman's primary duty was to produce children. Once weaned, the children were then raised by other adults—nurses, nannies, and instructors for the wealthy,

## OLDER MOTHERS

Between 1985 and 1995, the number of babies born to European and North American women between the ages of thirty-five and thirty-nine has risen 50 percent, while among younger women birthrates have declined. In France, the fertility rate for women over forty rose from ten in a thousand to fourteen in a thousand between 1979 and 1989—that's a 40 percent jump! In Paris alone, the percentage of pregnant women over forty tripled between 1990 and 1996. Of course, women over forty have always been having babies, but usually their last child. In fact, due to the absence of reliable contraceptives, more women over forty had babies a hundred years ago than do now. But what makes the past fifteen years different is the growing number of women who are having their *first* child after they turn thirty-five.

What are the differences between a forty-year-old and a twenty-five-year-old mother? Age is less of a factor than we think. Some people say that older mothers have less energy. This is not only untrue but older mothers are less likely to suffer from postnatal depression, extreme fatigue, and postnatal weight problems than younger ones. During pregnancy, they have fewer problems with nausea, they care better for their health, and they are more willing to accept change in their bodies. They also have fuller sex lives during pregnancy! They are better prepared for childbirth, and participate in it more actively. (However they are more at risk for disappointment if their birth experience is not flawless as their expectations tend to be high.) Once they return home, they usually have a larger network of friends to provide help and moral support. They may have the financial means to employ help with household chores. The baby's father is more likely to be involved and their life is generally more organized. Their postnatal physical problems (backaches and urinary incontinence, in particular) are similar to those of younger women.

It is also said that older women have more difficulty coming to terms with their new roles as mothers. It is true that after the arrival of a child, older couples tend to fall into a "traditional" division of labor: the mother looks after the house and children, while the father attends to the family's financial security. But studies show that in older couples where the woman is used to a certain independence through a professional career, the traditional roles are less in evidence. We find more "househusbands" and more women returning to work. In fact, 82 percent of women over thirty-five return to work after the birth of their first child, compared to only 32 percent of mothers under the age of twenty-five.

At the risk of overgeneralizing, we can say that studies show that older mothers are more patient and more relaxed, more emotionally mature, and take care of their own needs more readily. Two-thirds of women over forty who are pregnant for the first time worry that they will be extremely tired after childbirth, but report afterwards that they are pleasantly surprised by their energy levels. They do, however, admit that the arrival of menopause is harder with a small child or rebellious teenager at home.

Until 1981, half of all women over forty who became pregnant chose to abort their pregnancies. Today, women over forty have never been in better shape. They look forward to problem-free pregnancies and a positive experience of motherhood.

female relatives past child-bearing age and older sisters for the poor. In many families, children were put to work early so as to contribute to the household income.

The science of child development dates from the eighteenth century and appeared first in the book *Emile*, by the French philosopher Jean-Jacques Rousseau. This "instruction manual" on how to raise children was the first to distinguish between childhood and adulthood. Rousseau preached not only the importance of breast-feeding by the mother (at a time when most children were breast-fed by a wet nurse) but also the direct responsibility of the mother for her child's education. He was also the first to describe motherhood as a source of joy and satisfaction. As a result of this book's popularity among the affluent classes, women began to participate more actively in their children's upbringing. One hundred years later, raising children had become a full-time occupation for a growing number of middle-class mothers. The interest in science brought by the industrial revolution also touched the domain of child care, and mothering was viewed as a precise science with its own methods and rules. However, the industrial revolution also brought skyrocketing infant mortality rates to the working classes, whose health and living conditions were dire. In the late nineteenth century, some European governments finally launched "educational programs" for mothers that included threatening advertising campaigns to insure that state-sponsored recommendations would be followed.

By the early twentieth century, under the influence of Sigmund Freud and other founders of psychoanalysis, the mother was viewed as primarily responsible for the emotional stability of her child, and of the adult he would become. She would take the blame for the crimes or misdeeds committed by the son that she had raised. For the following half a century, dozens of theories appeared, many contradictory, claiming to be based on "science and progress" rather than on a mother's instinct and common sense.

After World War II, attitudes toward child care took another turn. Pediatricians such Dr. Benjamin Spock, psychologists such as Jean Piaget, and educators such as Maria Montessori insisted on the importance of stimulating and encouraging infants so that they would become confident, happy, and well-adjusted children. Toys were no longer simply to amuse, they also served an educational purpose.

Today we try so hard to be "good mothers" that we often sacrifice our own interests in order to concentrate solely on the needs of our children. The irony is that mothers have probably never been as "good" as they are now, yet never have they lacked so much confidence in their mothering abilities. We have such high expectations about childbirth, child development, and about our relationship with our partners that we are bound to encounter feelings of frustration and failure when things do not happen exactly as we envisioned.

Unfortunately, babies are not born with an instruction manual. Most new mothers are very anxious when their first child is born. (Pediatricians remark that mothers today are more anxious than they were twenty years ago.) Nevertheless, many women who were nervous about motherhood during their pregnancies discover that they are far less helpless than they had feared. And others, who read "everything" during pregnancy and who are "totally prepared," discover that they are overwhelmed when they find themselves home with a baby for the first time.

Trust your common sense and your intuition. Raising a child requires making spur-of-the-moment decisions. If there existed only one correct way to do things, we all would know about it by now.

Despite what certain child-care professionals may say in order to validate their role by making mothers feel incompetent, remember that it is a child's parents who really can make him happy.

Approach your new role as mother as you would approach a new job. If you were starting a new career, you would be given a training period, the time to learn new skills, a support network, time off, vacations, and professional recognition. Even newlyweds get a honeymoon! But not mothers.

We all know that when you start a new job, it's normal to feel a bit insecure. Becoming a mother is no different, and it's even more daunting because you've had no formal training beyond perhaps watching other mothers around you. Because most of us no longer live with an extended family, few of us have spent twenty-four hours next to a baby or a nursing mother. But society expects us to step easily into this enormous new responsibility—and to smile as we do it. So allow yourself the luxury of forgiving yourself for the mistakes you may make in the early days. Tell yourself twenty times a day: "I'm starting a new job, I need time to adapt."

We always try to do too much in the beginning. Our expectations tend to be set too high and since our self-esteem is involved, we easily become discouraged. Then we start to realize that we're doing too much, and we do a bit less. . . . There comes a time when we do just what we should, we find the answers by ourselves, and I think it's because we find them ourselves that they are the right answers. We all go through this cycle in order to stop fearing that we are bad, inadequate mothers. It's normal not to have unlimited, blind confidence in ourselves, but we should still have some confidence.

## Lack of Recognition

In our society, mothers suffer from an identity crisis. They receive none of the rewards granted to professionals: no big salaries, no drivers, no fame, and not even much social recognition. Raising children is a thankless job, performed behind the scenes by ranks of invisible women. It requires being on call twenty-four hours a day and a combination of a unique set of skills. Being a mother is a bit like the Chinese acrobat who juggles spinning plates at the ends of long poles: he is constantly running from one to the other so the plates will keep spinning and not shatter on the ground.

Even today, many people expect mothers to be utterly dedicated to their children and to quash any desire to develop other interests or tal-

## THE SECOND CHILD

Most women find it easier to raise their second child. Although they might be more tired, they are usually less anxious and less stressed. Many say that their second baby is easier. In general, mothers take their second child less often to the pediatrician than they did with their first baby, spend less time nursing, and are generally less worried about the baby's health and safety. For instance, they more readily go outdoors with the baby regardless of the weather. But the arrival of a second child can also bring new challenges. Each baby is an individual, with his own needs. This may be difficult to grasp at first, especially if the second child is very different from his older sibling. One piece of advice: if your relationship with your partner was deeply affected by the arrival of your first baby, take the time to consolidate your relationship before thinking of a second baby.

ents of their own. The Norman Rockwell image of a mother still prevails—comforting perhaps, but utterly lacking in individuality.

Yet, many people respect a woman only for her professional activities, not realizing how many skills are needed to run a household or to be a full-time mother. In a culture that measures success in terms of production, mothering is a flop: it produces nothing tangible, nothing that can be measured quantitatively. This is why some women feel the need to rush back to their jobs so as to "play a more productive role" in society.

Ironically, it is acceptable to look after other people's babies—as long as you get paid for it! Why do we consider women who spend the bulk of their time raising their children as "housewives," when that term clearly implies that the household, as unappreciated as it may be, is more highly valued than motherhood? Finally, what can we say about the working mother? Instead of criticizing her for dividing her time between two callings, instead of doubting her ability to handle both her professional responsibilities and her children, we should admire someone who performs "two jobs" for one salary.

All of this is a bit discouraging. But keep in mind that being responsible for the nourishment, protection, and care of a new human being can bring you an unequaled sense of joy and satisfaction. And even if the whole world seems to undervalue your work, the recognition of your partner and the love of your child will provide ample compensation for your efforts.

## Expectations Management

The disappointment that accompanies a lack of recognition is amplified if a woman's expectations are unreasonable. She may wish for a perfect, loving relationship with her baby, to whom she is completely dedicated. She dreams of an ideal life, of a baby who never cries because his every need is satisfied. Another woman may imagine that she will have organized her new life so well that she will have ample time for other activities. Disappointment is inevitable in both cases. The first mother wants to adapt her life entirely to the baby's needs, and the second mother wants a baby entirely adapted to her needs. The first fears she will not succeed in completely synchronizing her rhythm to that of the baby, she may end up resenting him. The second is afraid of falling in love with her child, of not controlling him, of producing a spoiled child who will dominate her life. This disillusionment can go on for

---

### IN CONCLUSION . . .

In the *New Mother's Body Book*, Jacqueline Shannon summarizes the major changes in perception of themselves and of the world which affect new mothers.

- Motherhood will make you much more aware of your own mortality.
- Motherhood will make you paranoid.
- Motherhood will change your idea of what makes for happiness.
- Motherhood will loosen your inhibition.
- Motherhood will change the way you view your parents.
- Motherhood may change what you look for in friends.
- Motherhood will change the way you feel about work.
- Motherhood will make you less selfish, less self-centered.
- Motherhood will change the way you view your community.
- Motherhood will change the way you think about the future.

years. The best way to avoid such disappointment is to remember that each baby is unique and rarely corresponds to the generalized descriptions we read in child-rearing books. Each has his own individual personality from birth. We all need to give up trying to mold our children in our own image.

## Additional Resources

Depression After Delivery (DAD)
91 East Somerset Street
Raritan, NJ 08869
800-944-4PPD
*www.depressionafterdelivery.com*

Postpartum Assistance for Mothers (PAM)
P.O. Box 20513
Castro Valley, CA 94596
510-727-4610

*Fragile Beginnings: Postpartum Mood and Anxiety Disorders* (Video)
Distributor: Injoy Productions
800-362-2082

*Heartache and Hope: Living Through Postpartum Depression* (Video)
Parent Development Centre
403-253-6722

*Postpartum Emotions: The Blues and Beyond* (Video)
Family Experiences Productions, Inc.
512-338-1318

# V

# The Couple

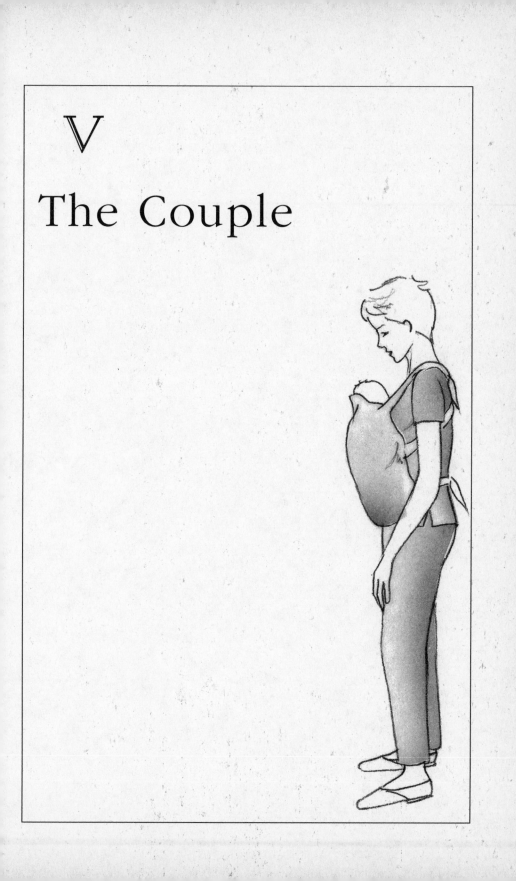

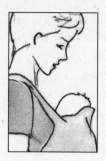

# 21

# The Couple Changes

In the United States, one in three marriages ends in divorce. In many cases, the separation occurs in the first two years that follow the birth of a child. Why is this?

The arrival of a baby, especially the first, transforms the relationship inside a couple. Three people now must share love, time, and energy. The exclusive nature of the couple's relationship comes to an end. Moral and material responsibilities grow, lives must be better organized, improvising becomes difficult, if not impossible, and the partners now must accept their interdependence. This realization can be overwhelming. In addition, if the parents are tired, they may be more irritable and find themselves arguing more frequently. New conflicts can arise on matters that both partners thought resolved, especially regarding values and important decisions such as education and religion. It is therefore not surprising to find that many women claim to be less satisfied with their relationship after the birth of a child.

Family history becomes important. The birth of a child causes both parents to look back on their own birth and childhood. Forgotten joys and sorrows are unconsciously reawakened. One parent may feel the need to repair past errors. He or she may also fear that a similar problem may repeat itself in the next generation. Even if the partner is not fully conscious of the reasons for his concern, it will affect his behavior, his moods, and reactions.

Another important factor will impact on the couple's new relationship. The woman will judge her partner according to a new criterion— his ability to be a "good father." With her newly acquired protective instinct, even the most relaxed, easygoing woman will become overcritical if the father does not live up to her expectations. If communication is good within the couple, if each partner feels that he can express his wishes and is attentive to the other's needs, there is no reason for the baby's arrival to become a crisis. But, if the woman does not know what her partner wants, or is not able to express her own desires, then couple's communication problems may intensify.

Unfortunately, this often happens. At first, the father feels left out of the magic bubble surrounding mother and child. He may feel sexually frustrated, clumsy, and useless around the baby, and he may not dare admit his feeling of disappointment. As for the mother, she may feel as though her new maternal responsibilities, physical pain, and emotional upheaval overwhelm her. Yet, she may not dare express her enormous need for affection and support.

The abruptness of these transformations is also an important factor. Most future parents simply cannot imagine just how much their world will change. Midwives note that few couples ask questions about the postnatal period during childbirth preparation classes. Nevertheless, the same protective instinct that makes a mother so demanding of her partner also compels her to do everything she can to create a harmonious environment for her child. For this reason, most women will do their best to overcome these difficulties, and the couple will emerge strengthened.

## When a Woman Becomes a Mother

A new mother's feelings toward her partner can be as varied as her feelings toward her baby; and they are not always positive. Frustration is once again quite common—usually due to unreal expectations. A number of other negative reactions are normal.

## A Feeling of Suffocation

Suddenly, a childless life seems wonderfully free and spontaneous as opposed to the constraints and responsibilities of motherhood. Even a stable partner relationship—now reinforced by the baby's arrival—may seem suffocating. Because she is now feeling vulnerable, the new mother may become uncommonly demanding, testing her partner's ability to be a "good father." Alone at home all day with the baby, far from the professional activities that give her a sense of individual identity, she may find herself dependent on the father for a breath of fresh, stimulating air from the outside world. But if the father feels detached from what is going on at home, while the mother is centered solely on her infant, the disparity between these two lives can cause tension within the couple.

Many women who had a stimulating professional life before becoming mothers are afraid of losing touch with the outside world, or of becoming "boring" by staying cooped up at home with a baby. Some 90 percent of couples surveyed go out less after the birth of a child, and this lack of outside recreational activity can quickly become constraining and frustrating for both the mother and the father.

## A Feeling That Everything Revolves Around the Baby

Having children satisfies a basic need for many women. But all women also need adult relationships. A child will never replace the man, the partner, and the husband. However, in situations where the woman feels misunderstood and undervalued, having a baby can be a way of asserting herself, of claiming an identity. The reasons for this are complex and often result from the mother's own childhood experiences.

Many women experience a decrease in sexual appetite after giving birth. This diminished urge can sometimes last for as long as two years. There is a pervasive myth (which many of us believe to a certain extent) that a child will fulfill us completely. Many writers, starting with Freud, have described the almost erotic relationship between mother and baby, to the exclusion of the father. However, in reality women are not entirely satisfied with their new "relationship." Indeed, one aspect of a woman's femininity is the fact that she is sexually desired by a man.

## Overemphasizing the Role of the Doctor

Sometimes, the obstetrician plays such an important part in the maternity process (especially in cases of assisted conception or of a problem pregnancy) that the baby's father is pushed to the side. When the ob/gyn is a man, the doctor's expertise, especially when compared to the new father's clumsiness or disinterest, glorifies him in a new mother's eyes. When the doctor must be involved to a great extent, it is important that the father be involved in the process as much as possible and not treated as a "fifth wheel."

## Making Motherhood Your Only Source of Fulfillment

Some mothers go out of their way to point out their partner's faults and clumsiness in handling the baby so as to reinforce their role as primary caregiver. Likewise, some men prefer to delegate all tasks concerning children to the mother (possibly as their father did with their mother). New mothers often have the impression that their husband or partner idealizes their maternal capabilities—a way of justifying their noninvolvement with the child. Thus, a woman's fears, fatigue, and uncertainties go unnoticed. She becomes resentful. His expectations are shattered. Women should remember that their partner cannot always guess the new mother's needs, especially if she is ashamed of her own doubts. Many fathers complain: "I don't know what my spouse expects of me. She has become completely mysterious." They think that their spouse will instinctively know what to do, while in reality, she feels as lost as he does.

Beware of judging your partner solely on his ability to care for the baby and "punishing" him if he appears inept or uninterested. Reducing your partnership to a matter of diapers and bottles is a serious mistake made by many new parents.

## Misunderstanding What the New Father is Going Through

It is a mistake to believe that the experiences of pregnancy and childbirth are destabilizing only for women. This myth reduces parenthood to a purely physical event and ignores the fact that becoming a father is equally unsettling and confusing. Every man has his own way of coping with this change; his initial reaction is not necessarily a sign of things to come in the future.

## When a Man Becomes a Father

A woman has the advantage of a progressive preparation for motherhood over the course of nine months. She carries the child not only in her body, but also in her heart and in her mind. Once the baby is born, she and the baby benefit from an extremely intimate relationship. The father-child relationship, however, is external and more abstract. He is usually less informed than the mother, rarely participates in initial baby care in the hospital, and does not often discuss baby issues with his friends and colleagues. Once home from the hospital, the baby and his supplies seem to take over the house. He is expected to stand close to the mother-child unit, but cannot enter into it; to instinctively take over all the housekeeping chores; and to have a sudden and burning desire to change diapers and give the baby its bath. It is hardly surprising then that he feels left out.

Many men do not express their emotions with ease ("grown men don't cry"), yet these feelings may be very intense at the birth of a child. New fathers may be just as unsure about living up to their partner's expectations, experience fatigue and loneliness, and cope with the same adjustment problems as women.

Though more short-tempered than usual, most women still expect their partners to provide affection and support. Many new mothers complain: "He didn't even say thank you." In a couple, there is always one partner who feels more confident than the other is. But here lies the dilemma: after childbirth, tradition expects the strong partner to be the man. Admitting to uncertainties is still seen by many as a sign of weakness.

Fathers also have spent nine months with an imagined child, and may also need some time to get used to the real one. If the mother finds it difficult to "adopt" her newborn even though she has had nine months to get used to a baby whom she has felt moving in her womb, imagine how much more difficult it is for a man to become a father.

## Mixed Feelings

In spite of his joy, a father can experience many mixed feelings about
the new baby:

+ He may feel threatened, now that all important decisions seem to be
  considered in terms of their impact on the baby. Older fathers may
  be especially worried that the baby will cramp their lifestyle.

+ He may be jealous of the woman's reproductive powers, which seem
  to bring her happiness and attention.

+ He may feel a strong burden of responsibility, as well as stronger
  professional and financial pressures to succeed, and thus provide
  adequately for his child. While this may make him feel important, it
  may also be a huge source of worry.

+ He may feel overwhelmed by his spouse's emotional dependence on
  him, particularly if the new mother is having difficulty recovering
  from the psychological aspects of pregnancy and childbirth.

+ He may be frustrated to find that his spouse appears to be perpetually engrossed in the baby and makes no time for him alone. This
  reinforces his impression that he is no longer important to her.

+ He may be alarmed by the baby's fragile appearance and not dare to
  touch him.

+ He may be angry about not having had a son and not show sufficient
  interest in his daughter.

## Misunderstood Reactions

These feeling may lead the father to react in ways that are easily misunderstood:

**He seeks refuge in his work.** This is a way of forgetting his problems by remaining in a world where he still has some control and feels
at ease. It is also a way for him to "procreate," to "give birth" to something himself. If he feels excluded from the mother-child relationship at

home, he may find comfort in his relationships with his professional colleagues.

**He lacks interest in the baby** and avoids caring for her (at least not in front of the mother). Often, if the father is alone with the baby, certain that no one is watching him, he relaxes and interacts with her.

Even if a father has not read and prepared for the baby's birth, he is perfectly able to care for a baby's basic needs. And if he does not put the diaper on quite the perfect way, it is not vitally important for the baby's well-being! The baby quickly becomes accustomed to the fact that every person has a different way of looking after her.

**He expresses an exaggerated interest in household accounts.** Our society still considers fathers to bear primary responsibility for the family's material needs. A father who experiences doubts about his parenting skills may concentrate on household finances as a way of escaping his deeper worries.

**He wants to take charge of everything**, as if he did not trust the mother's ability to care for the baby. This situation may occur in second marriages when the man already has older children but the woman is experiencing motherhood for the first time. Or else it may be the man's way of expressing his frustration at the woman's lack of confidence in her mothering abilities.

**He has nightmares, gets sick, or has an accident.** The baby's arrival might reawaken forgotten problems. By falling ill, he is reclaiming the attention that he resents no longer receiving. This type of behavior can also surface during his spouse's pregnancy.

**He suggests activities that are unrealistic** for a mother with a newborn, such as a night at the disco when his spouse is exhausted, travel to a place not suited for babies. Or he may frequently bring home large groups of noisy friends as a way to claim "his" territory. These are ways of "competing" with the baby by marking his place with "his" woman.

**His sexual desire for his spouse may greatly diminish or disappear.** This happens to many men during their wives' pregnancies. They are afraid of hurting the fetus, feel slightly offended by the physical changes in their wives' bodies, or are afraid of not satisfying the woman, whose sexual appetite increases during the second trimester of pregnancy. When the baby is born, they may have trouble accepting that their spouse is now both a mother and a sexual partner. Sometimes, new fathers actually make greater sexual demands, also as a way of reclaiming their partner.

**If the baby is difficult or has high needs, he can implicitly blame his spouse** and use this as an excuse for being home as little as possible.

**He wants to flee**, to establish a physical as well as an emotional distance between himself and the mother. He finds excuses to be away (work, travel, friends), or has affairs, to prove his independence from the mother-child unit which he feels is excluding him. This is usually a temporary phase. But if the father really does suffer from emotional immaturity, usually due to relationship difficulties during his childhood, he may panic at the idea of paternal responsibility, and actually run away.

Most of the time, these reactions are not signs of a permanent rejection but are an indication of the man's difficulty in adapting to his new role as a father. Bitterness and recrimination from the mother sets into motion a vicious circle of anger and escapism. A few simple gestures—such as trying to talk about something other than the baby, agreeing to going out once in a while without the baby, or planning a weekend getaway for the future—can ease the tension and show him that there is room for everyone.

## Father and Child

While some fathers fall back on the traditional stereotype that men are unsuited to handle small babies as a convenient escape from the more unpleasant tasks of baby care, other fathers feel the pressures of a new expectation that has grown in western society over the past twenty years. With the disappearance of the extended family and the increased professional involvement of women, men are now expected to become "father hens," sharing domestic chores, taking care of the older children, keeping the household running, and being sensitive to the mother's mood swings, while still maintaining their professional activities. A father today is caught between the weight of tradition and modern expectations.

Unfortunately, despite the few "super-fathers" we may encounter, most of us are likely to be disappointed if we expect our partners to undergo such a transformation. If the father feels that he is doing "woman's work," or if he is forced to join in on domestic work, he certainly is not going to enjoy it (even if he feels proud of himself afterwards).

Nevertheless, a father has two important roles to play which go far beyond the family's material needs:

### ✦ Provide a symbolic separation between the child and his mother.

As a child grows, one of the mother's important responsibilities is to teach him, gently but firmly, to become independent. This task, which can be quite painful, will be much easier if the father plays his role as the "separator." Child psychologists agree that it is vital for a "third party" to intervene in the mother-child relationship to keep it from becoming too exclusive so that the mother can rediscover her normal sexual desire for her partner. And this third party should be the father.

The father challenges the baby, often providing stronger sensations and emotion through the way in which he plays and communicates. For example, a father usually understands a toddler's babble less well than the mother and thus will require him to speak more clearly. It is with his father that a child explores and experiences new situations in a less frightening way. This paternal function is not necessarily linked to the biological function—it can be fulfilled by a man other than the child's biological father. But a child needs both routine activities (usually provided by his mother, the primary caregiver) and exposure to more intense experiences that generally come from other (often masculine) sources of stimulation.

### ✦ Provide a source of affection, support, and recognition for the mother.

Although it is sometimes difficult for a man to accept that his spouse is feeling vulnerable and overwhelmed, he can do more to help and comfort her than anyone else can. He can provide an objective "outsider's" perspective and cut through many of her worries to find a solution.

## Establishing a dialogue

It is important for a child to sense the importance of his father's role as companion to his mother, the person whose presence is necessary for his mother's happiness. In order to get through this difficult period as harmoniously as possible, the following tips may be helpful:

+ Don't become a prisoner of stereotypes. One major cause of postnatal tensions between a couple can be eliminated by avoiding the expectations implied in the roles of "father hen" and "perfect mother" and reestablishing frank, open communication. Don't hold back, tell your partner what you are experiencing; this can only bring you closer. Knowing your fears, doubts, and dreams can also reassure him, because chances are good that your partner feels the same worries you do. But be careful to tell him that your worries are not signs that you are rejecting him.

+ Try to respect his uncertainties. If your partner seems not to be interested in every last detail about the baby, this may be due to his insecurity about his role as a father or it may be an act of defiance against you or the baby. Do not force him to participate in the baby's care or make him feel guilty about his reluctance.

+ Try to understand the sensitivity of his situation. Ask yourself: "How would I react if I were only a spectator and not the main actor?" If you feel superior and show him contempt, it will only reinforce his feeling of unworthiness and will make him become more distant.

+ Recognize reality. Most men feel that their primary responsibility is in providing a sufficient income for their family and not in providing child-care services. Until we are truly liberated from traditional gender roles, there is little in our society to support a true egalitarian family model. Women may continue to work outside of the home, but their professional aspirations will remain secondary to their role as nurturer.

+ Ask him to fulfill precise tasks. A father cannot guess what is expected of him. Indicate exactly what you would like him to do so that he feels a sense of accomplishment in knowing he has satisfied your specific needs.

**A FEW TIPS**

Let the father take care of the baby alone, instead of forcing him to have a passive presence while you do all the work—which will only create a feeling of uselessness. Leave the room. Don't stand next to him commenting on the way he does things, or smiling condescendingly.

Avoid placing a hungry, crying baby in his father's arms unless it is to give him a bottle. Fathers tend to enjoy giving babies their bottles because they feel gratified when the baby appears satisfied.

Do not become fixated on the idea that the father has to take care of the baby "in order to bond." The father-child relationship is not necessarily built around the baby's physical needs. It blossoms and flowers in its own ways, which may be very different from what the mother could have imagined—and should remain their own secret.

♦ Make him feel needed. Show him that you need his love and support. Men often underestimate the amount of love they are capable of giving.

♦ Find time for yourselves as a couple. Babies instinctively know how to capture all the attention. Make time for your partner—and he must find time for you. The couple should not be overlooked for the child's benefit, because it is just as important to his well-being that his parents maintain a loving relationship.

## Common Stumbling Blocks

### On the Father's Side

New mothers usually are eager to rekindle their former harmonious relationship, to find themselves once again with the man they love and know. Fathers should try to avoid a few common blunders.

♦ Sleeping alone with the excuse that the mother must take care of the baby at night because you have to be in shape to go to work the next day.

- ✦ Refusing to get up in the middle of the night, even several nights in a row, to give the baby his bottle. Or giving the bottle but waking the mother up so she can change the diaper and put the baby back to bed.
- ✦ Complaining bitterly if dinner is not on the table or if a specific household chore has not been done. Nursing every three hours is exhausting and other aspects of daily life sometimes must give.
- ✦ Endlessly pushing the mother to "shape up." She needs time. Those extra pounds will eventually disappear but nagging about them will not help—particularly during the first three months after the baby's birth when it is useless to diet (see pages 140–141).
- ✦ Above all, the new mother needs tenderness, attention, affection, and understanding. She also needs to be appreciated in her new role as mother. This means making some concessions from time to time.

**If your spouse feels confident and happy thanks to you, you will be the first to benefit. So keep up your courage, and patience!**

## From the Mother's Perspective

What not to do:

- ✦ Be extremely demanding or on the lookout for the slightest slip the father may make when taking care of the baby.
- ✦ Demand that he be a "perfect father," which obviously does not exist, instead of accepting him as he is and giving him time to find his way with the baby.
- ✦ Be intolerant of the man's strange new attitudes, which are only signs of the upheaval he is going through while becoming a father.
- ✦ Reproach him, consciously or unconsciously, for being the source of pain of childbirth, and try to make him "pay for it."

## IN CONCLUSION . . .

The rule is the same for men and women, tolerance, goodwill, patience, and humor. It is a small price to pay for sharing the extraordinary adventure of bringing a child into the world.

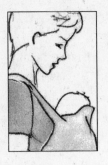

# 22

# A Little Patience:
# Sex After Childbirth

In many religions, sex is proscribed for forty days after childbirth. This period of abstinence actually has a medical justification: it takes six weeks for the cervix to heal. Some women may want to have sexual intercourse earlier than this, but we recommend as more prudent a gentle and gradual return to sex, at least six weeks after giving birth. Two-thirds of women find the first time they have intercourse after childbirth to be less than pleasant. A couple's sex life generally is less active even seven months after having a child than it was when they were expecting. In many cases it takes a good year to recover the satisfying sexual life the couple had before the woman became pregnant.

## Physical Impediments to Sexual Desire

During the first three or four weeks following childbirth, almost all women experience a period of physiological frigidity. The nervous connection between the brain and the sexual organs appears to be "anesthetized." The vagina is still dilated and the entire pelvic area is still tender. An episiotomy scar can remain painful for several weeks (and in some cases months—see below) and the internal bruising caused by forceps can also take a few weeks to heal. Other physical problems can get in the way of sexual pleasure:

+ Childbirth may cause some tearing in the blood vessels that line the vagina, thus preventing adequate engorgement and lubrication necessary for pleasurable sex.
+ The stretching of the vaginal muscles during childbirth coupled with the relaxing effect of the pregnancy hormones (see page 20) means a loss of vaginal tone and sensitivity that may last for several months.
+ The new, lower position of the uterus means that it is easier to bruise the cervix during intercourse.
+ If a woman is breast-feeding, the presence of the hormone prolactin (the "milk production hormone") may suppress her sexual desire.
+ Anemia can also cause frigidity, because it is often accompanied by a deficiency in folic acid, which is required for the proper transmission of sexual pleasure to the brain.
+ Other physical problems can also be obstacles: weight gain, a cesarean section, postnatal depression, and even sexual problems that existed before pregnancy.

Fortunately, for the vast majority of women, these problems are only temporary and resolve themselves. But they do illustrate the fact that a hasty return to sexual intercourse is not advisable. Furthermore, medical studies show that for several months after childbirth, two-thirds of women prefer to be cuddled and petted rather than to engage in more active sexual relations.

## Psychological Obstacles to Sexual Desire

During the postnatal period, women don't really have sex on their mind. For starters, they usually are not thrilled by their bodies' appearance. Exhausted and overwhelmed by the baby's demands, the thought of satisfying their partner can seem just too much. Furthermore, motherhood brings such a sense of physical, sensual contact with the baby that some women feel completely satisfied simply with cuddling the baby. In our society, physical contact outside of a sexual relationship is rare for most people before they have a child.

This lack of sexual desire is a sort of nature-made policing system, which ensures that the new mother will devote herself entirely to her baby. The dip in sexual interest does not constitute a loss of love, but women often worry that they are not fulfilling their "conjugal duties." Today's society puts so much emphasis on sexuality that we think we are abnormal if we go through periods of abstinence.

## The Fear of Physical Pain

Many women are simply afraid of the pain of sexual intercourse after childbirth, especially if they had an episiotomy. According to a British study, nearly 80 percent of women who had episiotomies had a painful first postnatal sexual experience; 19 percent admitted that intercourse was still painful three months after giving birth. Women who did not have episiotomies started having sexual intercourse again about a month sooner, and 40 percent of them reported having no pain.

Some women are tempted to blame their doctor for having "sewn them up too tightly." But, apart from rare surgical errors, the tightness of the vaginal opening is due to the scarring process.

Women may also be afraid of sex for other reasons: they fear that their cesarean or episiotomy scar will burst open, or that they might become pregnant again. And some women just cannot bear the thought of sexual intercourse as long as they are breast-feeding.

## The Wrong Moment

Between the ages of three weeks and three months, the baby generally cries more in the evening (just when his father returns from work!). Babies also have an astonishing ability to start crying just when their parents are beginning to get intimate.

New parents also may feel inhibited about having sex if another person (mother, mother-in-law, and baby nurse) has come to stay to help take care of the baby.

> ### IN SUMMARY . . .
>
> Do not begin having sexual intercourse again unless you want to and in any case:
>
> - Never before you have stopped bleeding (the risk of a cervical or uterine infection is great).
> - Never before the episiotomy scar has fully healed.
> - Never before the cesarean section scar has healed (twenty days).
> - Never without contraception.

## The Father's Attitude

Some fathers demand "their due," while others keep their distance for religious reasons, or just out of jealousy toward the baby. New fathers also can feel diminished sexual desire because they themselves are tired, or for more emotional reasons: some have a hard time recovering from the harrowing sight of their wife delivering a baby, and others may feel the woman who has become a mother is a holy, untouchable being. Other men, touched and moved by the birth, are attracted by the softness and voluptuousness of maternity.

Many women force themselves to resume their sexual life out of a sense of duty, so as to please their partner (above all if the father is showing signs of jealousy toward the baby), or even out of fear that he may "go looking elsewhere."

## Reclaiming Your Intimacy

### Transitional Sexuality

The first sexual encounter after giving birth should be a experience of "transition." A woman's feelings and her erogenous zones have changed, her body is still fragile. Gestures that excited her before may leave her cold now. It may be necessary to invent new caresses and new positions. Knowing how to rekindle sexual passion may be a difficult task for a man if his wife does not guide him. Some women are offended that their husband is asking for sexual relations while they are still deeply engrossed in maternity.

Sensuality can be recovered however before the resumption of sexual relations. In this way, the steps are gradual: caresses and massages are a good beginning, before moving on to a clitoral orgasm, and then penetration.

## Privacy

Most of the time, a new mother does not feel very comfortable about herself. It is unlikely that she will be the one to take the first step. But she can try to "break the routine" in order to create an atmosphere that encourages intimate relations. Often, it is after a first dinner for two, or after going out without the baby for the first time, that the couple rediscovers itself.

If you have other children at home, and you have not yet thought about putting a lock on your bedroom door, it might be the right time to do so. You can then be alone without worrying about a child's intrusion, and be more relaxed about finding your way back to sexual pleasure. Do not be embarrassed about explaining to your children that Mommy and Daddy need to be alone sometimes, and that they need to be together to love each other.

## Breast-feeding and Sexuality

For many women, breast-feeding alone satisfies their desire for intimacy (moreover, nursing contributes to vaginal dryness, and lengthens the reaction time to sexual stimulation). It may delay the resumption of a sex life resembling what it was in the pre-pregnancy days. Conversely, if a woman is unable to breast-feed, she may vent her frustration by unconsciously refusing to feel sexual pleasure.

Some fathers are jealous of their wife's intimacy with the baby, and may try to impose sex as a way of reaffirming their position. But for other women, nursing brings such a sexual blossoming that her libido, and the couple's sex life, is reinforced.

## When the Woman Feels Ready for Sex

+ Feed the baby just beforehand, so as to have some peace and quiet. And put the baby in another room.
+ Nurse or pump your milk, before beginning foreplay, so your breasts will not be engorged.
+ Keep a towel nearby because oxytocin, the "love hormone," also makes milk flow.
+ Lubricate your vagina (lubricants are widely available in drugstores and pharmacies without a prescription). The drop in estrogen levels can make the vagina walls dry until your menstrual period returns.
+ Avoid taking a bath just before making love, because that further dries the vagina.
+ Make foreplay last longer than usual to give the vagina time to lubricate itself.
+ Penetration may be painful initially, but the pain will disappear when the penetration is deeper. It is therefore important to take care during penetration (by lubricating, advancing gently, and adjusting your position). Once he is inside, the man must be attentive to the woman's signal before continuing.
+ The classical "missionary" position is the least comfortable after giving birth, especially if the breasts are full. The penis rubs against the rear wall of the vagina, just at the level of the episiotomy scar. The shaft must be as vertical as possible so as not to hurt the cervix which is still sensitive, and it must push against the side of the vagina that is opposite to the episiotomy scar. After a cesarean section, pressure on the belly will be almost unbearable.
+ If the woman is on top of the man, she will have more control over the depth and direction of penetration. This position also allows her not to feel dominated.
+ If the delivery was difficult, do not re-create the same position: on your back with your legs lifted. It could bring back bad memories and "kill" your desire. Some women feel they are "traveling backwards" when they resume sexual activity. It will take patience and gentleness to recover, little by little, the confidence necessary to feel real sexual pleasure again.

## If Pain Persists

It can take several months to recover and heal from a difficult delivery—and some symptoms may never fully disappear, even if they are psychological. If sexual activity continues to be painful (the medical term is *dyspareunia*) after several tries, you should definitely consult your doctor. Deterioration of sexual intimacy is today the cause for 70 percent of divorces. It is an important problem, and you should not be content to wait and hope that it will disappear with time.

Urinary incontinence during physical exertion does not necessarily mean there will be problems with sexual activity, but it is better to warn your partner: it could be embarrassing during pelvic movements and at the moment of orgasm.

After an episiotomy, you might feel a sort of knot at the base of the vagina. To avoid pressure and friction during penetration, the pelvis must swing upwards (place pillows beneath your lower back and pelvis) so that the penis rubs the upper part of the vagina and the base of the clitoris.

In case of extreme pain, it is useful to examine your vulva with the help of a small mirror. A small black or red mark is probably a stitch that was not removed or absorbed by the body. The doctor can remove it in a matter of seconds.

A red scar that is swollen or oozing can be a sign of infection. You should contact your doctor immediately for an appropriate treatment.

If the pain is very localized and sexual activity is made impossible by the pain, there may be a *neuroma* (a ball of nerves) at the site of the episiotomy. In serious cases, this can be removed surgically.

Sometimes, the vaginal muscles close involuntarily and resist penetration. This phenomenon, called *vaginismus*, indicates that the body is not ready to resume sexual activity that includes penetration. If this persists, it may be advisable to consult a psychotherapist (preferably a woman).

# VI

# A Full
# Recovery

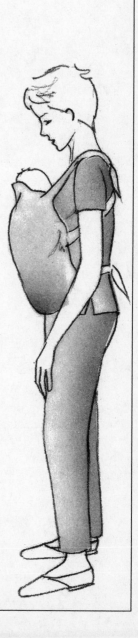

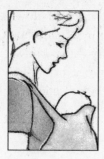

# 23

# First Things First:
# The Pelvic Floor

## The Importance of the Pelvic Floor

This chapter concerns those two-thirds of new mothers who, when asked about their pelvic floor, respond, "Everything's fine thank you"—yet who probably may not even know where it is located, or what purpose it serves or, most importantly, how much it has been weakened by pregnancy and childbirth. What follows is a warning call for all new mothers to take notice about an important part of the body that does not receive enough attention from pregnancy books, the media, or even the medical community. Toning the pelvic floor is your first step toward recovery.

As the population ages, as greater numbers of women have children over the age of forty, as women become increasingly athletic later in life, we will be faced more and more with problems such as urinary incontinence and prolapsed organs. Already today, more than half of us will suffer from a bout of incontinence at some point in our lives. The sanitary pad and adult diaper business is thriving, but meanwhile one woman in three does not know how to contract her pelvic floor muscles correctly (she will tighten her buttocks, raise her pelvis, or push out her stomach, but not "lift and squeeze" as described below). Two out three women cannot distinguish between the three main muscle groups of the pelvic floor (anal, vaginal, and urinary—also known as the *levator ani* muscles). Yet each group's tone may be very different from the other. And most women do not contract their pelvic floor muscles before sitting down or lifting a heavy weight.

## A Number of Myths Surround the Pelvic Floor

◆ Urinary incontinence and prolapsed organs are a problem of old age. *False*. Fifty-five percent of all women will experience urinary incontinence at some point in their lives, half of them before the age of fifty.

◆ Incontinence is a fact of life, too humiliating to discuss with your doctor. *False*. On average, women wait seven to nine years before discussing a leakage problem with their doctor. Yet the problem often can be solved with a few sessions of specialized physical therapy!

◆ It's no use worrying about your pelvic floor until you have given birth for the last time. *False*. It's after the second baby that the pelvic floor suffers the most. Many cases of incontinence during menopause are due to a pelvic floor weakened by childbirth.

◆ My doctor will tell me during my postnatal checkup if I need to do something about my pelvic floor. *False* (at least much of the time). Most gynecologists are trained but frequently fail to test the pelvic floor muscles. It is you who knows that you have a problem with urinary or anal leakage, or who feels water dripping out of your vagina a few minutes after a bath, or who no longer feels as much pleasure during sex. It is up to you to discuss these issues with your doctor and request a prescription for specialized testing or therapy.

◆ I need not worry about my pelvic floor if I have had a cesarean section. *False*. Although the baby will not have come down the birth canal and distended the pelvic floor, pregnancy itself has a major impact on these muscles: pregnancy hormones cause all of the body's muscles and ligaments to loosen, much greater weight bears down on the pelvic floor, and the bad posture of many pregnant woman stretches these weakened muscles in the wrong direction.

## What You Can Do

Understand the anatomy of the pelvic floor—its role in supporting the abdominal organs, the mechanism of the sphincters, the importance of toned pelvic floor muscles to a satisfying sex life.

Understand the concept of "closure"—before birth, we prepare our bodies to open up but we forget that closing up also requires effort. Yet, this process is essential to becoming a woman once again, now that we are holding the baby in our arms and no longer in our bellies.

Make the effort to exercise the pelvic floor muscles regularly according to the prescriptions given on pages 296 and 297 of this book. And, if necessary, do not hesitate to seek professional help to solve a problem through physical therapy.

Integrate prevention into your daily lives by knowing how to move, breathe, and carry loads to protect the pelvic floor.

## Lift and Squeeze: A Brief Review of Pelvic Floor Anatomy

The network of muscles between our legs is composed of two parts: one stretches like a hammock from the pubic bone to the tailbone. This is the actual pelvic floor (the network of levator ani muscles) which lines the bones of the pelvis like a floor ending in a point with the anal canal. The floor bears the pressures of all the genital and digestive organs piled above it. The second part of the network consists of three groups of muscles (the sphincters) that surround the three openings of the pelvic floor: the urethra, the vagina, and the anus. They are composed of two or three layers. Thus, when the pelvic muscles are contracted, two things happen: the pelvic floor muscles lift and the sphincter muscles contract. This notion of lifting while squeezing is fundamental—one hears too often of squeezing only.

The *pubococcygeal* muscles perform numerous functions: supporting the weight of the organs, holding back gas, excrements, and urine, balancing the spinal column, and contributing to pleasurable sexual intercourse. In this respect, the pelvic floor muscles can be compared to a trampoline, flexible enough to absorb the body's moving and shaking, yet sufficiently strong to keep the internal organs in place. This is possible through the interaction of two types of muscle fibers:

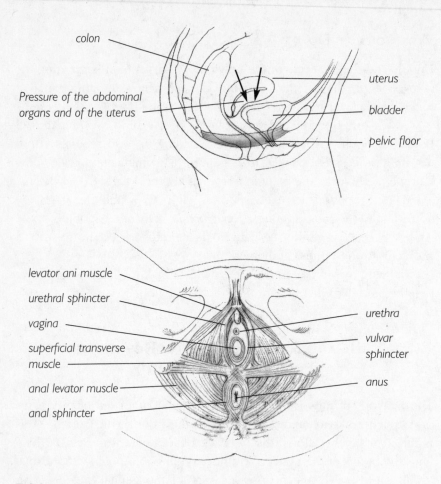

colon

Pressure of the abdominal
organs and of the uterus

uterus

bladder

pelvic floor

levator ani muscle

urethral sphincter

vagina

superficial transverse
muscle

anal levator muscle

anal sphincter

urethra

vulvar
sphincter

anus

**Pelvic anatomy**

"slow fibers" (70 percent of the levator ani muscles) which provide
strength and tone, and "fast fibers" which provide instant, powerful
contractions when there is a sudden change in pressure—such as when
you try to stop urinating in midstream. All of these muscles intersect,
forming a fibrous knot in the area between the vulva and the rectum—
precisely the point at which the pelvic floor is cut in an episiotomy.

Because an impressive number of blood vessels and nerves are
located in the pelvic floor, its good tone and health are important to the
entire pelvic area.

# What Affects the Pelvic
# Floor Muscles?

The strength and tone of the pelvic muscles is dependent on a number of factors—the impact of pressure from the abdominal organs, proper or improper breathing, good or bad posture, as well as specific conditions such as constipation, pregnancy, or damage incurred during childbirth.

## The Pressure of the Abdominal Organs

All the abdominal ligaments and muscles must work together to resist the forces of gravity, of daily life (walking, carrying heavy loads, coughing), and of exceptional pressures (obesity, respiratory illnesses, vigorous sports). The quality and tone of the muscles and ligaments that hold and support them determine the proper placement of the abdominal organs. They are able to stretch gradually fairly efficiently. But when subjected to a sudden trauma (such as during childbirth), they are unable to adapt. For example, during a jump, gravity doubles the weight of the abdominal organs at the moment of impact. Thus if a woman jumps into the air, her uterus will now exert a pressure of twice its actual weight on the pelvic floor. This explains why so many female athletes who practice high-impact sports suffer from urinary incontinence.

## Breathing

Shallow and incorrect breathing, which causes tension in all the body, directly affects the pelvic floor. This is why proper breathing is so important in childbirth, particularly at the moment of delivery, in order to minimize damage to the pelvic floor muscles.

## Posture

Because the pelvic floor is attached to the pelvic bones, their position will determine how the pelvic floor muscles are pulled and stretched. If a woman's posture is bad, the muscles around the edges of the pelvic floor may be pulled too tightly while the sphincters in the middle are too loose.

## Constipation

Bearing down too hard will compress the rectum and push down the pelvic floor. Over time, the pelvic nerves (which are important to feeling sexual pleasure) will be stretched and lose sensitivity.

## Pregnancy

Pregnant women tend to arch their lower back to compensate for the increased weight they bear in front. But to regain their balance, they then roll their shoulders forward. The result is not only back pain but also a distension of the pelvic floor muscles, which are pulled along their edges and too loose around the sphincters.

During pregnancy, the weight of the uterus increases by twenty- to thirty-fold. As it grows, the uterus then pushes the bladder downward. Furthermore, the ligaments and muscles that normally hold up the genital and digestive organs are now weaker under the effect of pregnancy hormones. Thus the pressure is great on a pelvic floor, which itself is already strained. This explains why many pregnant women experience problems with leaks of urine or gas.

## Childbirth

This is probably the greatest single source of stress on the pelvic floor muscles. Actually, the pelvic floor recovers after the first child in most women. It is after the second birth that most women do not recover.

The pelvic floor muscles will be stretched and distended by childbirth, no matter the baby's position, the way in which his mother pushes, or even how well she has prepared for delivery. Following any vaginal birth, the pelvic floor loses about 50 percent of its muscle tone. Nevertheless, the chance of damaging these muscles can be greatly reduced with proper preparation: stretching exercises, perineal massage, and techniques to coordinate pushing and exhalation are all helpful preventive measures.

## The Following Factors Usually Have a Harmful Impact on the Pelvic Floor

+ When the expulsion stage of labor happens too fast (the baby comes out "like a champagne cork"), the baby can pull the reproductive organs down with him and cause major complications—large tears, muscular lesions, eventually a prolapsed uterus. Fortunately, obstetricians today are better able to reduce the damage caused by such overly rapid births.

+ When the woman is made to lie in the lithotomy position (flat on her back, feet up in stirrups), the baby's head may compress the urethra and strain the pelvic joints. Women are usually asked to breath in, hold their breath, and push. This movement increases the intrauterine pressure and also makes the pelvic floor muscles tense and rigid. Some practitioners recommend that if the woman pushes as she breathes out, her knees folded back at a 90-degree angle, the abdominal muscles will work more efficiently and the pelvic floor muscles will remain supple.

+ Other childbirth procedures can have a damaging effect on the pelvic floor: certain major maneuvers to turn the baby, pushing on the woman's stomach to expedite delivery, or stimulating uterine activity with large doses of oxytocin.

+ If the tailbone has been displaced by the baby's head (occurs in 10 percent of all vaginal births), the pelvic muscles to which it is anchored will then be pulled down and back. This can be very painful.

+ If the episiotomy has been badly repaired, this can cause tensions within the pelvic muscles.

## The Pelvic Floor and Sexuality

How well your vagina returns to its normal dimensions after childbirth is linked to the muscle tone of the pelvic floor. If the vagina remains distended, there will be less sensation during sex. Sometimes, the vagina makes embarrassing noises (as it passes gas) during sex or exercises such as a shoulder stand. Another symptom of vaginal distension is noticing water dripping out a few minutes after a bath.

Forty-two percent of women with a urinary incontinence problem also experience some degree of sexual dysfunction: a pressing need to urinate during or immediately after intercourse, urinary leakage during sex, or painful intercourse. Incontinence therefore can have a harmful effect on a relationship.

As we have seen, 30 to 45 percent of new mothers who have had an episotomy complain that sex is still painful even three months after childbirth. Sometimes, this is due simply to a weakness of the pelvic floor muscles.

Fortunately, all of these cases can be treated effectively with specialized physical therapy, especially if treatment is begun soon after childbirth.

# Urogenital Problems

Most urogenital problems (which affect one in three new mothers) usually disappear within six weeks after childbirth. But if the delivery was very traumatic or if the pelvic floor is particularly weak, these problems may persist until properly treated by a specialist.

## Symptoms of Urogenital Problems

- ✦ Urine leakage during a sudden contraction of the abdomen, such as when laughing, coughing, sneezing, jumping, or being frightened.
- ✦ A feeling of pressure or weight in the pelvic area, pulling, or a backache.
- ✦ Vaginal gas or water dripping out of the vagina after a bath, or a feeling of vaginal distension.
- ✦ Chronic constipation.
- ✦ Frequently passing rectal gas, liquids, or feces.
- ✦ Painful intercourse or a lack of sensation, or inability to achieve orgasm.

Though these symptoms may all be linked to a weak pelvic floor, each may require treatment by a different specialist: gynecologist, urogynecologist, gastroenterologist, neurologist, proctologist, or urologist. One should nevertheless understand the relationship between the various organs involved.

## Urinary Incontinence

Medical research on the causes and prevention of urinary incontinence has made enormous strides in the past fifteen years. But as is often the case, a better understanding of the problem has also meant an increase in statistics. Today, it is said that 54 percent of women will experience some form of urinary incontinence at least once in their lifetime . . . often during the postnatal period.

Unfortunately, incontinence is still a subject that we consider embarrassing and concerns a part of the body we avoid discussing in public. This denial remains the greatest obstacle to an effective dialogue between women and the medical community.

## How Does it Happen?

When functioning normally, the two kidneys filter our blood and transform the waste materials into urine that flows continually, drop by drop, into the bladder. Once the bladder is filled with about 250 milliliters of urine, a signal is sent to the brain that makes us feel the need to urinate. Two muscles (the *sphincters*) control the bladder's opening into the *urethra*, a tube that is about two inches in length that leads to an external orifice. One of the sphincter muscles plays a passive role in keeping the bladder closed (just like other involuntary muscles of the body such as the stomach), but relaxes during urination. The other one can be commanded at will. When we decide to urinate, the bladder contracts automatically under the influence of an involuntary reflex. To stop urinating, the muscle must not only compress the urethra but also pull it upwards. This process, which occurs about seven times a day (but hopefully not at night), requires perfect coordination between the bladder and the sphincter.

Normally, when the bladder experiences a sudden strong abdominal pressure (cough, laugh, sneeze, jump, or high-impact exercise), it immediately sends the sphincters a message to close tightly. But if the sphincters have been damaged, they cannot respond effectively.

If the pelvic floor muscles are distended or weak, the voluntary sphincter can no longer clamp down properly on the bladder opening. Thus, when a sudden pressure occurs (laugh, sneeze, cough, jump), a few drops of urine may escape. This is known as *stress incontinence.*

If the bladder has been distended or injured during childbirth, it might begin sending conflicting signals to the brain, such as requesting to be emptied when it is not yet full.

If the bladder is no longer well suspended in the pelvis and falls too low, the sphincters will have difficulty in performing their appointed tasks.

If the urethra has been damaged, the sphincter muscles will no longer open effectively and a problem of urine retention may occur—possibly leading to bladder distension or infection.

Although many cases of postnatal urinary incontinence will resolve on their own, the problems may reappear and worsen after each pregnancy and especially at menopause. For this reason, it is extremely important not to ignore these symptoms and to consult a doctor the first time that they occur.

## What You Can Do

In cases of persistent incontinence, your gynecologist will first will prescribe a number of tests: as a group the are know as urodynamic testing. He/she may refer you to a urogynecologist or a urologist for this. The tests consist of:

+ Urethral close or leak point pressure, which measures the muscle tone of the urethra and the sphincters.
+ Cystometry that uses gas or water to measure variations of pressure as the bladder is filled.
+ Pelvic or urethral spinctometry, which evaluates the compression ability of the muscles at rest.
+ Urethral Pressure Profile that quantifies pressure levels at different points on the urethra.

### Based on the Results Obtained, Various Treatments Are Available
+ Medication to increase the strength of the involuntary muscles and thus help keep the bladder closed.

- Specialized physical therapy to tone the pelvic floor, which may include electric stimulation and biofeedback (see pages 298 to 299).
- Surgery, in serious cases, when therapy has not worked. Support problems can be corrected through surgery, but sphincter tone and strength can only be increased through exercise.

## Anal Leakage

During the postnatal period, many new mothers experience some form of anal leakage (gas, liquids, or feces). These problems are due to a weakened anal sphincter usually caused by a difficult birth that distended the pelvic floor muscles and overstretched the pelvic nerves, or by a general weakness of the area (such as occurs after repeated close births). If the anal sphincter was torn during childbirth, the nerve endings may also have been damaged and specialized physical therapy is highly recommended. A proctologist can measure the condition of the anal sphincter with instruments similar to those used by a urologist.

Unfortunately, most women are reticent to discuss urinary incontinence—and are even more embarrassed to reveal an anal problem. Yet most of the time it can be solved or at least greatly improved with a few sessions of specialized physical therapy.

## Organ Prolapse

The suspension action of ligaments and the supportive action of muscles hold our abdominal organs in place. When one side of this system weakens, the organs are pulled downwards by gravity and may no longer function correctly.

### Causes of Organ Prolapse

- Childbirth, especially if the baby is very large, or if the delivery was long and difficult.
- Resuming strenuous activities or carrying heavy loads too soon after childbirth.

+ Professional activities requiring many hours of standing or carrying of heavy loads.
+ Respiratory problems (especially chronic coughing or sneezing).
+ Chronic constipation (pushing too hard).
+ Certain hormonal upheavals that affect muscle and ligament tone (especially menopause).

If the front ligaments are too loose, the bladder will fall against the vaginal wall (and can be felt as a hard ball from within the vagina). This is known as a *cystocele*. If the ligaments that hold the bladder "neck" in place are weakened, the bladder will have a tendency to curl inward, pushing the vagina down toward the vulva (external genitalia). This is a *cystourethrocele*. If the rear ligaments that hold up the cervix debilitate, the uterus will fall into the vagina. In extreme cases, the cervix can be felt at the vaginal opening. This is a *uterine prolapse*. And if the ligaments that hold up the colon are distended, the rectum will push against the rear of the vagina, making it difficult to defecate. This is a *rectocele*. Several of these forms of prolapse can occur simultaneously, effecting urination, bowel movements, and, of course, sexual function.

## Warning Signs

+ A feeling of heaviness in the lower abdomen.
+ A sense that "something is falling" inside.
+ Lower back pain.
+ Difficulty in keeping a tampon inside the vagina.
+ Pain or numbness during sexual intercourse.
+ Urinary incontinence (in two-thirds of cases).
+ A need to urinate frequently.
+ Hemorrhoids.
+ Pain on defecating.
+ Gas or bowel incontinence.

## What Can Be Done

Specialized physical therapy can go a long way toward restoring muscle tone in mild cases. Even in more serious situations when surgery is required, physical therapy is essential to ensure that the pelvic floor is as strong and supportive as possible. Furthermore, since surgery will

---

## PROLAPSED ORGANS

### Herbal Remedies

- Essential oil of Evening Primrose and essential oil of Palma Rosa (2 drops on a lump of sugar or with a spoonful of honey) are excellent toners of the urogenital system.

### Homeopathy

- One dose of Arnica 9C and 1 dose of Causticum 7C or of Sepia 9C taken twice a day.
- You also may want to consider the following:
  - If you feel abnormal heaviness or a dragging sensation: Sepia 200C, three doses in 24 hours.
  - If your intestines or your bladder feel paralyzed (especially after a cesarean): Opium 5C three times a day.
  - If the prolapse is accompanied by sleeplessness or numbness, Helonia 4C three times a day.
- In cases of prolapse of the rectum or of injury to connective tissues: Ruta 200C, 3 doses in 24 hours.

---

almost inevitably cause a loosening of the urinary sphincter, it is useful to undergo a few sessions of therapy to strengthen the sphincter in the two or three weeks before the operation.

Specialized physical therapy for the abdominal muscles and the sphincters requires about three months of diligent exercises and careful monitoring thereafter. One useful exercise to practice at home (while lying on your back, with your feet propped up on a coffee table or sofa cushions) is the "elevator" described on page 298.

Surgery may be required in serious cases of prolapse. The decision to operate depends on the patient's age, whether she plans to have more children, the degree of functional difficulties caused by the prolapse (such as incontinence or painful sex), and potential future problems that may occur. Surgery should only be considered after a women has completed her childbearing.

# Toning and Strengthening the Pelvic Floor

One of the most important aspects of post-pregnancy recovery is to "reconcile" yourself with your body—especially the genital zone. This process helps ensure the return of a good-quality sex life.

## Do It Yourself

### *During Pregnancy*

As we have seen, the influence of hormones (especially during the first two trimesters) and the pressure of the baby on the uterus tend to weaken the pelvic floor and make toning exercises (*kegels*) less effective. Nevertheless, this is the time to ensure that you know how to contract your pelvic floor muscles correctly without using your stomach or buttock muscles. Since childbirth will have such an important impact on the pelvic floor, it also is important to learn how to relax and how to push properly. There exist various forms of prenatal exercise techniques to suit each expectant mother. Some include perineal massage, which midwives find effective in reducing the possibility of tearing during delivery. Most importantly, pregnant women should watch their posture, especially when carrying loads, and learn how to contract their pelvic floor muscles before any demanding movement. If you already have problems with urinary incontinence during pregnancy, especially during the first two trimesters, now is the time to discuss an appropriate postnatal therapy with your doctor.

### *In the First Five Days Following Childbirth*

The exercise described on pages 79 and 81 help tremendously in alleviating postpartum discomfort by stimulating blood flow to the pelvis and thus speeding the healing process. As we discussed, they will also have a beneficial psychological impact by helping you overcome the feelings of emptiness and lower-body numbness that often follow childbirth.

### *Once Home, Between Six Days and Three Weeks After Delivery*

You should continue with the exercises on pages 79 and 81. During this period, it is critical to watch your posture and to avoid lifting anything heavier than your baby because your ligaments are still distended and your uterus is four times its normal weight.

### Three Weeks After Childbirth

You should be able to hold a contraction for three to four seconds (with a long-term goal of ten seconds). Learning to relax (for twice the length of the contraction) is equally important.

## How to Contract the Pelvic Floor Muscles Correctly

Lie on your back, without underwear, knees bent, legs apart. Hold a hand mirror in front of your vagina. Squeeze and lift your pelvic floor muscles. You should see a tightening of the muscles between your anus and the vaginal opening (if you place a finger on this zone, you will feel the ascending motion). If you are contracting correctly, the anus puckers and withdraws. Try coughing while you hold the contraction. Can you do it?

The most common errors are to squeeze the stomach muscles, buttock muscles, the inside of your thighs, or clench your fists, your toes, or your jaw at the same time. You can test how well you manage to relax the rest of your body by placing a hand on your stomach. You should not feel any movement while you are doing your exercises.

### Breathing

Breathing should be independent of these exercises. It is not particularly important to train yourself to contract your pelvic floor muscles as you inhale and to relax as you exhale since you don't want to automatically let go when your cough or sneeze. However, it is important to focus on breathing properly and deeply during these exercises to ensure an adequate supply of oxygen to the area. Deep breathing also "massages" the lower abdomen and eases the entire zone. The more you activate the pelvic area, the better the blood will circulate and help to heal and eliminate toxins.

### Holding Your Urine Midstream

This well-known exercise calls for you to stop urinating in midstream by contracting the muscles of your urinary sphincter. It is recommended in many maternity wards and pregnancy books because it is colorful and easy to understand.

Today, however, urologists and physical therapists specializing in uri-

## THE ELEVATOR

Toward the sixth week after childbirth, you can try the following challenging exercise. Imagine that your pelvic floor is an elevator that goes up four floors (the top floor being your waist). Go up a floor. Wait a second. Then go up another floor. Wait a second. Then go up again. Hold and continue until the top floor. Then go down again, a floor at a time. When you have perfected this, try going down to the second floor only and then back up again. Smile. Don't tense your shoulders or your buttocks.

nary incontinence have issued a warning: stopping your urine in midstream should only be used as a test of pelvic muscle tone and no more than once or twice a week (never more than once in the same day). Even if you cannot achieve it on the first try, do not try again. Most women cannot stop their urine midstream until four weeks after childbirth.

When attempting this test, you should hold the urine stream for at least ten seconds. Most importantly, only try this exercise as you begin to urinate or else there may not be enough urine left for the bladder to empty itself completely. If urine stagnates in the bladder, it can cause infections. The test is only useful if performed in tandem with other pelvic floor exercises—it will not strengthen the other two sphincters (anal and vaginal).

Regular exercise, good posture, and prevention (contracting the muscles before sitting down or lifting a load and knowing how to push in case of constipation)—all of these should be part of every woman's routine during her entire life.

## Specialized Physical Therapy for the Pelvic Floor

While many women can do these exercises at home, a prescription from a gynecologist or urologist for specialized physical therapy may be necessary if:

+ Early signs of an impending prolapse have been detected.
+ The distance between your anus and you vulva is less than one inch.
+ You are required to stand all day at work.

- ◆ You carry heavy loads or you spend more than two hours a day in a car.
- ◆ You exercise more than five hours a week.
- ◆ You experienced urinary leakage during pregnancy (especially during the first and second trimesters).
- ◆ Your mother or grandmother suffered from incontinence.

**Be sure to choose a physical therapist with specialized training or a registered nurse who has been trained in the treatment of incontinence.** Given the psychological connotations of pelvic floor muscle rehabilitation, it is important to select a therapist and an approach with which you feel comfortable or else you will not be sufficiently motivated to complete your course of therapy.

In order to test the tone of the pelvic floor muscles, the therapist must be able to gauge their ability to contract, their closure capacity at rest, and their resistance to fatigue. This can be done manually by inserting into the vagina two slightly bent fingers in a lubricated examination glove. The therapist will then ask the patient to push against the fingers. Although this evaluation method relies on the perceptions of the individual therapist, it does allow for considerable subtlety in differentiating between the various parts of the pelvic floor. For example, after an episiotomy incision, muscle tone can very greatly from one side of the pelvic floor to another.

Following the initial evaluation, the therapist may use a number of tools such as passive electrostimulation (sending an electric current through a probe to stimulate the vaginal muscles), biofeedback, or cones (weights inserted into the vagina), as well as manual exercises to help restore pelvic tone.

*Please note*: The pelvic floor muscles will not fully regain their tone as long as you are breast-feeding since they are very sensitive to hormonal levels in the body. If you do undergo specialized physical therapy during the postnatal period, it is important to conclude with a few sessions after you get your period back.

It also is useless to start a course of physical therapy if your tailbone (coccyx) was displaced during delivery (which happens to one in ten women who deliver vaginally). If you feel great lower back pain or pulling on your episiotomy scar, it is important to see a therapist (preferably a manual therapist—chiropractor or osteopath, see pages 10–15), who first will put everything "back into place."

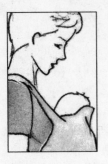

# 24

# A New Body Image

## Your Weight

As we have seen in the previous chapter, it is essential to tone the pelvic floor muscles before launching into any other post-pregnancy exercise program. Once this is accomplished, you can focus on recovering the size, shape, and tone of the rest of your body.

For most women, returning to their pre-pregnancy state is a major challenge that is difficult to achieve without some form of outside assistance: signing up for a training program at your gym or joining an exercise class (especially one designed for new mothers) will give you the motivation needed to achieve your goals.

The speed at which each woman recovers (and hopefully improves on) her shape depends on her individual metabolism—the rate at which she burns calories, at which her circulatory system supplies her body with oxygen, and at which her lymphatic system rids the body of toxins. Then, almost every woman needs to combine dieting with exercise to slim and tone.

## When Can You Start Losing Weight?

During pregnancy, most women gain twenty-five to thirty-five pounds on average. Immediately after delivery, the mother is about fifteen pounds lighter: the baby accounts for seven to eight pounds, the placenta for one or two pounds, the amniotic fluid and lost blood for another one to two pounds. Within the first two weeks, another five to ten pounds in excess fluids are dropped through urination. The process then slows. For example, the uterus takes about eight weeks to shrink from a weight of about 2.3 pounds at delivery to about two ounces. But some women still look seven months pregnant for several weeks after childbirth.

Let's be realistic: the great majority of women really begin to lose weight and get their shape back about six months after childbirth—even if they started dieting at six weeks! So don't bother with a strict diet or exercise program (other than the exercises described on pages 119–121) until the baby is three months old—and only if your are no longer breast-feeding and the baby is sleeping for seven hours a night. This does not mean, however, that you should not watch what you eat by following the guidelines on page 135–41.

## What Should You Weigh?

Weight can be evaluated in a number of different ways. Do not confuse the weight you wish you weighed with your potential weight (which is a function of heredity and of our weight history), with your ideal weight (that at which the risk of cardiovascular disease is the lowest), or with your fitness weight (that at which you feel your best).

The best way to set your goal is to calculate your body mass. This standard is used by many health professionals but requires using the metric system. First convert your height from inches to meters (multiply by .025). Then convert your weight from pounds to kilograms (multiply by .45). Then divide the weight by the height squared. If the result is:

+ less than 18, you are probably too thin
+ between 18 and 20, you're slim
+ between 20 and 25, your weight is ideal
+ between 25 and 30, you have a few pounds to loose
+ more than 30, you should see a nutritionist.

## WEIGHT LOSS

Vitamins $B_6$ and $B_{12}$, as well as zinc and vitamin E act as hunger suppressants by balancing brain chemistry. Most mothers are deficient in vitamin $B_6$. You should consume between 15 and 50 milligrams per day. It can be found in beef, pork, chicken, fish, potatoes, soy, avocado, barley, quinoa, and cauliflower. Vitamin $B_{12}$ not only plays a vital role in controlling hunger but also helps fight fatigue and anemia. It is difficult to meet the recommended daily allowance for zinc of 12 milligrams even if you consume 3,000 calories per day, since only about 20 percent of the zinc we eat actually is absorbed. You may find that taking these as supplements is helpful while you are trying to lose weight.

### Homeopathy
- To eat less: Pilosella TM or Nicotinum 5C.
- To keep your spirits up while you are dieting: Ignatia 5C or Escholtia T.
- To avoid eating sweets: Pulsatilla or Anacardium 5C.
- To calm hunger pangs: Oligostim Zinc.
- If you were already a little overweight before your pregnancy and you like rich foods: Antimonium Crudum 5C.
- If you eat too fast and have a tendency to feel blue: Ancardium Orientale 7C.
- If you feel drained, tired, and frequently want to eat small quantities of food: Amonium Carbonicum 5C.
- If you lose weight when you work but gain weight when you are not busy: Calcarea Carbonica 7C.
- If you are often cold and have a slow digestion: Graphites 7C.
- A daily boost when dieting (4 granules of each):
    Morning: Anacardium 7C (reduces hunger).
    Noon: Sulfur 4C (to help your digestion).
    Evening: Antimonium Crudon 4C.
    Before bed: Natrum Sulf 4C.

### Herbal Remedies
- Prepare an herbal tea with equal quantities of Blackberry, Artichoke, Dandelion or Blackberry, and Green Tea.

### Aromatherapy
- Mix equal parts of essential oils of Clove, Rosemary, Peppermint, Caraway, and Cypress. Take 1 drop of the mixture on a sugar cube or with a teaspoonful of honey three times a day.

If your result has not changed, just stick to the dietary recommendations in Chapter 10.

If your result has changed from your pre-pregnancy days, but still lies between 20 and 25, you are still at your ideal weight—but you may feel better if you shed a few pounds by watching your diet and by toning your body.

If your result is now between 25 and 30, you probably should diet, aiming to lose about one or two pounds a week.

If your result is above 30, you will find it much easier to achieve your ideal weight under the guidance of a dietitian or a nutritionist.

## How to Diet

Simply limiting your food intake to 1,500 calories a day, which means reducing by a third the recommended calorie allowance during pregnancy, will lead to weight loss. Within these limits, you can vary the foods you eat, even indulge yourself from time to time, then stabilize your intake at about 1,800 to 2,000 calories a day while losing five to eight pounds a month.

Don't forget the saying "the more you diet, the more you gain weight." Starving yourself at 1,000 calories a day sends the body into a state of want. It reacts by drawing energy from the muscles. But a new mother's muscles are already weaker than normal. It is therefore useless to weaken them further. The body sends out an alarm signal and begins to store more fat while increasing the sense of hunger. This explains why it is so difficult to maintain a "starvation" diet. In other words, losing weight is a question of balance.

In Chapter 10 on post-pregnancy nutrition, we recommended that all new mothers be especially careful about their choice of foods. This principle also is important when dieting because the origin of calories is as important as their quantity. Metabolizing proteins consumes more energy than metabolizing carbohydrates. But while carbohydrates and proteins supply the same number of calories (4 calories per gram), fat contains more than twice as many calories per gram! Eating smaller, more frequent meals and snacks increases the rate at which calories are burned and promotes the regular flow of blood fats (triglycerides) inside the fat cells in the tissues of the body.

# Exercise

## How and When to Start Exercising

As you begin to recover from childbirth and to feel more autonomous, it is important to start thinking about your body image. Many new mothers tend to neglect their appearance in the weeks following childbirth—but dress their baby up in lovely outfits. The baby is in the limelight, and the mother slips back into the shadows. The sad truth is that when faced with flabby, overweight bodies, most women are discouraged even at the prospect of the effort they will have to make to recover their shape and muscle tone. But you must remember that fat can only be removed from fat cells when it is burned in muscles as energy. It also is extremely important to show your partner and your children that, although a mother now, you are still a woman. Taking pride in your appearance is one way to preserve your identity as an individual.

Some women who miss the attention they received during pregnancy unconsciously want to keep their round belly. Others feel so overwhelmed by motherhood that they lack any interest in appearing attractive to their partner for several months. Some will even "test" their partner by making him wait. As described on page 265, the postnatal period can be very trying for the father who feels neglected, even rejected, while the mother is engrossed in her baby.

Fortunately, most women wake up one day to realize that a strong adult relationship is also important to their well-being. This moment usually coincides with an urge to take control of their life again, to get out of the house and—often most importantly—to wear their old clothes!

Nevertheless, it is important to remember that childbirth inevitably transforms the body and that we must learn to accept this changed appearance. All pregnant women will typically gain about 8.8 pounds on their hips, thighs, and buttocks. Fortunately, your postpartum metabolism will burn off some or maybe most of it in the weeks and months after childbirth. But the recovery process may seem frustratingly slow. A recent study shows that only 22 percent of women have lost all their pregnancy weight gain six weeks after childbirth. A further 37 percent have lost it all by six months. But 41 percent still carry extra weight well into their baby's first year. Remember, it takes five to six

## WHEN TO START EXERCISING

### First Six Weeks
- Pelvic floor and abdominal exercises (page 297).
- Walking (one hour a day—not pushing a baby carriage)—132 calories per hour burned.
- No dieting allowed.

### At Six Weeks
- Swimming (unless you are still bleeding)—462 calories per hour burned.

### At Two Months
- Aerobic walking (3 mph)—180 calories per hour burned.

### At Four Months
- Bicycling—300 calories per hour burned.
- Competitive swimming—960 calories per hour burned.
- Tennis—564 calories per hour burned.

### After One Year
- Running—528 calories per hour burned (not recommended after three children).

months for the ligaments to recover their elasticity and tone (and therefore for the abdominal organs to be properly suspended again), up to one year to get your waist back, and up to six to seven months on average for your weight to normalize. It is tempting to ignore those last five pounds and simply to buy clothes in a larger size. But if you plan to have more children, do you really want to put on five pounds each time? Furthermore, the body's metabolism slows after age forty and these pounds will become that much harder to shed. (See page 301 to determine your ideal weight.)

Of course, we all hear about models and actresses who get their figure back within weeks of giving birth. What the press does not reveal is the cost required—not only in financial terms (personal trainers, dietitians, and figure-sculpting equipment, even surgery) but also in terms of the potential future health problems resulting from dieting and exercising too soon after childbirth.

## The Importance of Cardiovascular Training

Losing weight without simultaneously exercising is in fact just eliminating water and muscle. The body will protest by stockpiling fat. And fat can only be burned by working the muscles . . .

Toning and strengthening the body's muscles, which is essential after pregnancy and childbirth, should be accompanied by cardiovascular exercise (exercise which increases the heart rate) approximately four months postpartum after checking with your doctor (except for walking and swim-

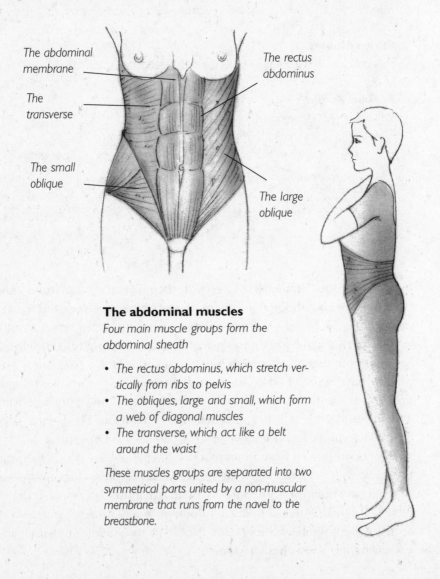

The abdominal membrane

The rectus abdominus

The transverse

The small oblique

The large oblique

**The abdominal muscles**

*Four main muscle groups form the abdominal sheath*

- *The rectus abdominus, which stretch vertically from ribs to pelvis*
- *The obliques, large and small, which form a web of diagonal muscles*
- *The transverse, which act like a belt around the waist*

*These muscles groups are separated into two symmetrical parts united by a non-muscular membrane that runs from the navel to the breastbone.*

ming, which you can start on your own as soon as you stop bleeding). Fat will not be burned and eliminated without increasing the heart rate.

Walking for forty-five minutes to an hour on a regular basis is the best postpartum exercise. It is the cheapest way both to lose weight and to restore your emotional equilibrium.

## The Abdominal Muscles

They can be compared to an elastic tube located under the skin that is anchored to the backbone, the ribs, and the pelvis—a little like a Victorian corset. Two long muscles, the *rectus abdominus*, lie on top of the tube, stretching from the ribs to the pelvis, like two suitcase straps. As they contract, they pull the ribs to the pelvis.

As a group, the abdominal muscles form a wall that protects the internal organs, ensures the correct alignment of the pelvic bones (along with the buttock muscles), supports the spinal column, allows for bending and twisting in all directions, and helps the body in all expulsion movements (coughing, sneezing, defecating, giving birth).

In addition to the rectus abdominus, the *obliques* form a web on either side of the abdomen, and the transverse muscles run in horizontal layers at the deepest level. However, in the middle of the stomach, there is only one layer of muscles. This explains why the belly area is the most flexible, but also the weakest and most vulnerable part of the abdomen.

On average, the rectus abdominus are thirteen inches long. During pregnancy, they will stretch 50 percent more to about twenty inches while waist size doubles. Right after giving birth, you may notice two bulges separated by a hollow in the middle of your stomach, especially when you contract the muscles. These are the rectus abdominus, which have been pushed apart by the baby and by the effort of delivery. Dur-

### TO RECOVER A FLAT STOMACH YOU MUST . . .

- Not gain more weight during pregnancy than the amount recommended by your doctor.
- Return to your ideal weight after childbirth (see page 301 to calculate your ideal weight).
- Have good posture.
- Work daily on strengthening the oblique.

ing the first four days, you may be able to insert two fingers between them. Little by little, this space will narrow but abdominal muscle tone cannot be restored without exercise. After childbirth, the abdominal muscles will never again be as strong and therefore will more easily be pushed out again by another baby or even a bowel movement. Therefore, it is extremely important to strengthen the stomach muscles for more than aesthetic reasons. They can be trained to look flat again.

Poor abdominal muscle tone is the cause of:

+ **Back pain**. A flabby stomach is not only a soft stomach; its muscles lack tone and are probably overextended. The stomach organs are pulled forward, the lower back overarches, and the front of the pelvis tips down. All of these abnormal tensions contribute to back pain.

+ **Pelvic floor distension**. If the belly is bloated, the pelvic floor muscles will almost certainly also be distended. If the abdominal muscles are weak, posture probably is bad and tensions will not be distributed properly along the pelvic floor.

+ **Emotional distress**. There is also an important psychological advantage to abdominal exercises, as they will help a new mother "rehabilitate" the empty space left by the baby.

Abdominal work is therefore important—but not just any exercise, not just any time.

It is essential first to strengthen the pelvic floor. Strong abdominal muscles will push down on the intestinal organs. If the pelvic floor is too weak to provide the necessary support, a prolapse may ensue (see pages 293 to 295). And if a prolapse has begun (but may be as yet undetected), working on the abdominals will only aggravate the situation.

In the first days after childbirth, you can begin strengthening the pelvic floor with a number of very gentle breathing exercises and abdominal movements.

Do not undertake any exercises in the standing position until the pelvic floor has regained its tone. And if you delivered by C-section, we recommend doing all abdominal exercises lying down on the floor with your knees bent for the first eight months after childbirth.

While working on the obliques (whose job it is to pull in, lift and squeeze the stomach while supporting it), be sure to avoid exercising the rectus abdominus, which will make the stomach stick out and push the bladder and uterus downwards.

Oblique muscle exercises may seem boring but they are the only way to recover a flat stomach. Later on, you may also wish to work on the internal thigh muscles (the abductors) as well as deeper abdominal muscles and those that control the diaphragm. As a final step, you can add contractions of the buttocks, thighs, lower leg, and ankles.

Full sit-ups, "scissors," "bicycling," and other exercises done while lying on your back with both your legs up also are to be avoided.

## Posture and Your Back

Though the back may appear sturdy, it is the part of the body where emotional troubles express themselves in the form of physical problems. This is why the back muscles often are hard and tense. Indeed, most people need to work on relaxing the back before attempting to strengthen it.

After exercising the abdominal muscles, it is important to stretch the back since a tense back will diminish the beneficial effect of working on your stomach. If you are exercising with a trainer or in a class, be sure that back stretches are included in your sessions.

The key to good posture is the position of your feet and of your pelvis. Take a few minutes to stand in front of a mirror and try the following test. If you answer yes to one of these questions, ask a fitness professional to help correct your position.

- Are your shoulders at the same level?
- Do your shoulders fall forward (or are they comfortably pulled back)?
- Is your chest sagging (or held up)?
- Is your abdomen pulling downward?
- Does your lower back curve upward like a duck tail?
- Are your hips tense? Do they fall forward?
- Are your knees locked? Do they lean inward?
- Are your hands, fingers, or your toes tense?
- Is your jaw tense?
- Do you feel bloated or heavy?

When walking in the street, look at your reflection in shopwindows and correct your posture. As we have stated several times throughout

**A FEW TIPS**

Exercising in a heated pool is ideal for women recovering from childbirth. Working in warm water allows for a maximum effect with minimum effort. The buoyancy of water reduces stress on the body's joints (especially the lower back vertebras), which have been taxed during pregnancy, and allows for a gentler workout. The pressure of water against the body stimulates blood and lymphatic flow, while massaging the muscles.

this book, bad posture causes harmful tensions on the pelvic floor muscles and on the ligaments that support the abdominal organs. Breathing is hampered, so the body's energy does not circulate freely.

## The Breasts

As they do not contain any muscle, the breasts are much less well equipped to fight the effects of gravity. They are extremely sensitive to hormonal fluctuations and their size changes considerably during pregnancy. After childbirth, they lose their firmness and will only begin to get their shape back after the menstrual cycle resumes. Unfortunately, in some cases, the mammary gland atrophies (with or without breast-feeding) and the breast remains "empty."

Nursing will not harm the appearance of the breasts. It is the increase in volume of the breasts during pregnancy and gentleness of the weaning process that are the crucial factors in determining your breasts' appearance after pregnancy and childbirth—not nursing. Quite the opposite: breast-feeding helps restore their balance but the effect will be noticeable only after one year.

A good bra is essential and should be worn night and day (even if you are not breast-feeding) after childbirth.

## The Legs

After pregnancy some women find that their legs appear skinny (especially around the calves). In fact, the fat has moved elsewhere. The solution: plenty of walking and climbing stairs.

This last aspect of your recovery may seem frivolous to some, but is

---

## TONING YOUR BODY

### Herbal Remedies

- To improve circulation and limit the spread of cellulite: massage the area with Santelle Sisatique.
- To improve the shape of the bust: Essential oil of Geranium contains plant hormones that act in a similar fashion to human hormones. Massaging the bust and the area under the breasts twice a day with the following mixture of essential oils can help restore a shapely bust: 16 drops Ylang-Ylang and 9 drops geranium in 50 ml of a base oil (except Jojoba).
- To tone the thighs: Essential oil of Juniper has a diuretic action that firms and tones. Essential oil of Cypress acts as an astringent. Jojoba oil helps to eliminate fat and excess toxins. Massage the thighs with a mixture of 10 drops Cypress, 10 drops Juniper, and 5 drops Lavender in a base oil that is at least 50 percent Jojoba.
- A few drops essential oil of Juniper in the bath are also helpful.
- All of these plant extracts are effective only if massaged assiduously into the affected areas over a period of several months.

---

nevertheless important. Many women on a diet find that their face and breasts appear thinner but that they are not losing an inch from their hips. Fortunately, a number of methods exist to "shape the body"— some more effective than others. Their goal should always be to stimulate the body to improve the flow of oxygen to its tissues, and to drain away excess fat and toxins. We have selected several approaches that are worthwhile if undertaken in tandem with healthy eating habits, good posture, and an exercise program.

## What Is Cellulite?

It's the engorgement of the lymphatic system and the soft tissues in a specific part of the body (especially the pelvic area, knees, thighs, and ankles). Fatty deposits (*adipocytes*) are imprisoned in a network of watertight compartments filled with a solution of water, salt, and hormones that cannot be evacuated. The external symptoms of cellulite are skin that looks like an orange peel or "grains of rice" (the trapped fluids press against the skin, forming little bumps), as well as tenderness (as opposed to fat, which does not hurt).

Primarily bad circulation, nervous disorders, or a hormonal imbalance causes cellulite. But there are also numerous secondary causes to cellulite: constipation, a weak liver (especially if too much sugar is consumed), bad digestion, or even bad posture, which leads to poor circulation.

Pregnancy hormones favor the appearance of cellulite by causing water retention and poor circulation.

In order to treat cellulite, two simultaneous actions are required: dislodging the fatty deposits and eliminating the waste. Any treatment method that does not include both actions cannot be effective.

*Liposuction*, a form of plastic surgery, is the most radical means of eliminating cellulite definitively by vacuuming the fatty deposits. However, if the circulatory, lifestyle, or hormonal problem (which caused the cellulite to appear in the first place) is not resolved, the cellulite will reappear in other parts of the body.

In addition to the methods described above, the following steps should be taken to fight cellulite:

+ Changing your dietary habits, such as drinking plenty of fluids, reducing your sodium intake, increasing your protein intake (lean meats, fish, chicken, shellfish), as proteins have an anti-swelling effect.
+ Restoring the body's hormonal balance if a problem exists—some women find that the birth control pill causes cellulite to appear.
+ Treating nervousness and anxiety (preferably through natural or alternative therapies).
+ Doing abdominal exercises to tone the muscles and fight constipation.
+ Taking a light diuretic, not more than once or twice a week.

## Varicose Veins

Our circulatory system contains a network of arteries (which transport "new blood," rich in nutrients and oxygen), as well as veins (which carry used blood to the heart so that it can be purified and once again replenished with oxygen). Though larger and more plentiful than the arteries, the veins have thinner walls and are therefore capable of greater dilation and contraction. Two major systems of veins cross the body: the first, embedded in deep tissues, carries 90 percent of the used blood while a more superficial network carries the remaining 10 percent. The two networks are connected by a system of smaller "one-way" veins that allow the blood to flow only from the surface to the depths of the body. Blood moves through the veins with each heartbeat, aided by muscular contractions and the impulse given every time we take a step.

Inside the veins, a series of valves pushes the blood forward with the pumping motion of the heart. They must therefore be tight and toned to keep the blood from stagnating or flowing backwards. If the surface veins become enlarged, or if their valves no longer work efficiently, blood stagnates or flows in the wrong direction. The veins then become extremely visible and cause tingling or cramps. This condition is known as varicose veins.

The "varicose illness" (its medical term) is hereditary and congenital. It lasts a lifetime: it can be treated effectively but never cured. Seventy percent of those afflicted are women. Phlebologists (doctors specializing in vein problems) often are able to predict future varicose vein sufferers by looking at the legs of a patient's parents.

Because hormones have a major impact on venous tone, varicose veins often result from hormonal disturbances such as those caused by pregnancy, birth control pills, menopause, or hormonal treatment. The impact of pregnancy hormones on the elastic tissues of the body also causes the veins to dilate (one in four women gets varicose veins during pregnancy). Their walls become thin and are easily distended by the increased amount of blood that flows through the body of a pregnant woman. Varicose veins can appear during the first trimester of a first pregnancy, especially if the problem runs in the family. Despite what is commonly thought, 70 percent of varicose veins appear before the sixth month of pregnancy.

As the uterus grows, it pushes the vena cava against the backbone, thus hampering blood flow. If a pregnant woman stands for long periods of time, her added weight and the effect of gravity further slow blood circulation, thus worsening the situation (two extra pounds of weight in the stomach represents an added pressure of eight extra pounds on the lower body's venous and lymphatic systems).

Varicose veins tend to appear first on the lower edge of the buttocks, on the outside of the thighs and legs, on the back of the knee (where they are particularly painful), on the edge of the foot and ankle, and even on the outer lips of the vagina (from where they disappear within a few hours after childbirth, but may resurface at the next pregnancy). In other cases not related to pregnancy, they can also appear on the esophagus, the vocal cords, or the abdomen.

After childbirth, the veins may shrink back to their normal size and recover their tone, thus permitting the valves to function efficiently once again. But if the veins remain dilated, their valves will never recover completely. This explains why varicose veins tend to worsen with each pregnancy (even if they seemed to disappear completely after the first baby).

## Causes

As we have seen, varicose veins are principally due to a hereditary weakness of the venous system. But they can also be exacerbated by heat and sun (which increases venous dilation), crossing your legs (which hampers circulation and constricts one of the body's main surface veins), a sedentary lifestyle (the veins will not benefit from the pumping effect of walking), too much standing (gravity hampers the performance of the valves), or a weight gain of more than twenty pounds during pregnancy.

There is little to be done about heredity, which is the primary contributing risk factor for varicose veins. However, the following preventive measures should be tried:

+ Raise the end of your bed.
+ Wear support hose.
+ Never bathe in water that is hotter than 99°F.
+ Avoid under-floor heating.
+ Take vitamin B supplements.
+ Avoid spicy foods.

## Exercise

With each breath, the rise and fall of the diaphragm will aid in pumping blood through the veins and up to the heart. Making the diaphragm work hard through cardiovascular exercise will help overcome stagnation in the veins.

## What the Doctor Can Do

Most women wait until their varicose veins have become very unsightly or painful before seeing a doctor. Many put off a consultation until they have had "all their babies." Yet a number of remedies exist to alleviate the problem. Since varicose veins cannot be cured and require annual maintenance, it is better to begin treatment sooner rather than wait for the situtation to worsen.

**Sclerotherapy:** If only the small surface veins ("spider veins") are affected, the doctor can treat the condition by injecting them with a chemical that will cause the walls of the vein to swell and fuse together. Once the circulation stops, the vein will cease to function and will eventually be re-absorbed into the body. This procedure is relatively cheap and simple, but must be repeated regularly (about once a year) as veins will regenerate themselves.

**Surgery:** If the varicose illness affects either of the two large superficial veins of the legs (*the saphenous veins*), it should be removed. After determining the size of the affected area through a Doppler scan, this procedure involves extracting ("stripping") the damaged section and tying off ("ligation") any affected branches.

Fortunately, there are many more blood vessels in the body than required to meet our circulatory needs. But veins do grow back.

# Acknowledgments

This book was first gestated in France thanks to the advice and support of fifty-five specialists:

In particular, Dr. Daniel de Pariente, OB-GYN, my medical advisor; Monique Jolly-Poulain, physiotherapist and psychotherapist; and Agnes Mignonac, dietician.
    As well as:

**Acupuncture**: Dr. Jean-Michel Frey
**Dermatology**: Dr. Monique Pelisse
**Gynecology-sexology**: Dr. Marc Ganem
**Gynecology-psychology**: Dr. Sylvain Mimoun
**Fitness instructors**: Susan Barlier, Josette Calmeil, Patrick Joly, Mrs. Mars, Françoise Weidmann
**Homeopathy, herbal medicine, and nutritional therapy**: Dr. Syliane Koch, Dr. Bernard Saal, Dr. J-M Tétau
**Manual therapies**: Jean-Michel Eté, Dominique Guetta, José Kunstler, Laurent Serpaggi, Marie-Claude Vidal
**Naturopathy and aromatherapy**: Ghislaine Gerber, André Nahum, Dr. Christian Perez
**Nurse-midwives**: Chantal Birman, Alice Grainger-Gasser, Maria Knerr, Benoît Legoedec, Christine Michel, Anne-Marie Mouton, Valérie Niel, Dominique Olivier, Anne-Marie Pierret, Geneviève

Ravillon, Séverine Ravillon, Marcelline Retailleau, Anne Siri, Gudule Taffin-Reneaud, Margot Theiux, Dominique Trinh-Dinh
**Nutrition:** Dr. Eva Mimoun, Dr. Patrick Sabatier
**Periodentistry:** Dr. Sylvain Altglas
**Physiotherapy:** Philippe Bonnan, Heide Bosc, Catherine Casini, Véronique Lancereau, Roland Leclerc
**Phlebology:** Dr. Claudine Sicard
**Proctology:** Dr. Jean-Marc Gélinet
**Relaxation therapy:** Dominique Ravarit
**Urology:** Dr. Odille Cotelle-Bernède, Dr. Jean-Marc Duclos, Dr. Yves Thébaut

Among the three hundred women who were willing to share their postnatal experiences with me either through my questionnaire or in interviews, my thanks in particular to Alina Barrowcliffe, Corinne Bauer, Mathilde Coste, Amanda Fischer, Ileana Giesen, and especially Annick Mareuse, who turned my "franglais" into proper French.

Two fairy godmothers tended to the rebirth of the book in English, Elizabeth Wise and Melissa Greenwald, while Mary Dowd Struck supervised its adaptation to American medical practices with the help of Margaret Howard, PhD, Director of the Postpartum Depression Unit, and Dr. Debra Myers, uro-gynecologist, both at Women and Infants Hospital, Providence, RI.

# Index

abdominal muscles, 306–9
  exercise for, 307–9, 312
  pelvic floor and, 287, 289, 295, 297,
    308
abdominal pain, 85, 125
absentmindedness, 96, 231, 242
acetaminophen, 1, 31, 40
acini, 159–60
acne, 70, 128, 130
acupuncture, 3, 8–10, 239, 241
after-pains, 28–31, 70–71
alcohol, 191
allergies, 156
alternative remedies, 2–15
*Alternative Therapies for Pregnancy
    and Birth* (Thomas), 3–4
alveoli, 159–60
anemia, 25, 58, 96, 128, 146, 179, 219,
    275, 302
  diet and, 136–37, 141
  weakness due to, 52–53

anesthesia, xv, 6, 46, 49, 89, 123
  childbirth side effects and, 53–54,
    56–57, 62–66
  in c-sections, 53, 63, 68–71
  emotions and, 207, 213
  physical aftereffects of, 63–64, 69
  psychological effects of, 65
  urination and, 42
anger, 209
  couples and, 265–66, 268
  depression and, 218, 220
  perfectionism and, 245, 247
  postnatal depression and, 231, 236
antibiotics, 1, 74, 123, 126, 224
  breast-feeding and, 178–83
  for postpartum complications, 85–87
antidepressants, 240
anti-inflammatories, 1, 31, 40, 60
anus, 32, 45–46, 48, 58, 79
  childbirth side effects and, 58–61
  genital organ care and, 33–34

anus (cont'd.)
  pelvic floor and, 284–86, 288, 290,
    293, 297–98
anxiety, 15, 198, 201, 211, 256, 312
  child care and, 254
  depression and, 221, 225, 231, 234
  stress and, 228
areolae, 159, 165, 168, 175–76
aromatherapy, xvi, 3, 7–8, 239, 241
  for after-pains, 31
  for baby blues, 215
  for breast milk production, 172, 180
  for childbirth side effects, 54
  for constipation, 48
  for depression, 225
  for episiotomies, 40, 124
  for fatigue, 113
  for infections, 127
  for postpartum complications, 86, 90
  for skin, 129
  for weight loss, 302
aspirin, 6, 53

babies:
  carrying of, 115–16
  enjoyment of, 99
  physical appearance of, 201
baby blues, 21, 198, 210–15, 234
  causes of, 211–15, 217
  lifestyle changes and, 95–96
  symptoms of, 210–11
  treatments for, 6, 14, 214–15
baby-sitters, 101, 103–4
Bach Flower Remedies, 8, 215
back, back pain, xiv, 141, 288, 308–10
  breast-feeding and, 164, 170
  causes of, 55–57
  emotions and, 218, 229, 232, 239,
    246, 252
  exercise and, 308, 310
  infections and, 125
  lifestyle changes and, 96–97
  pelvic floor and, 290, 294, 299

  in postpartum complications, 86–87
  posture and, 115–17, 309–10
  treatments for, 11–12, 54–57, 61, 72
  varicose veins and, 313
  see also spine
barrier contraceptives, 144–45
beans, 137–38, 224–25
bicycling, 305
birth canal:
  caring for, 31–33
  see also episiotomies
birth control pills, 144–45, 192, 313
bladder, 64, 69, 96, 124–25
  exercises and, 83, 309
  genital organ care and, 28–29
  pelvic floor and, 286, 288, 291–92,
    294–95, 298
  in postpartum complications, 85, 88
  in urination, 42, 44
bloating, 45, 48, 75, 136
blood, blood pressure, blood vessels,
    blood tests, bleeding, 19–20,
    22–28, 49–50, 82–85, 87–90,
    120–23, 143–46, 161–62, 291
  body image and, 301–3, 307, 310–15
  breast-feeding and, 159, 161, 174, 177
  causes of, 88
  childbirth side effects and, 53, 57–63
  in c-sections, 68, 76
  diet and, 134, 136–37
  emotions and, 122, 197, 208, 215,
    218–19, 224
  exercise and, 49, 79, 307, 310
  genital organ care and, 28, 30, 32,
    35–39
  from gums, 132
  hygiene and, 43, 121
  lifestyle changes and, 96, 102
  pelvic floor and, 286, 297
  postnatal visits and, 146
  postpartum complications and,
    84–85, 87–90
  primary, 88–89

recovery process and, 23–27
secondary, 89
sexual intercourse and, 275, 277
treatments and, 2, 9–15, 59, 90, 122–23
varicose veins and, 11, 57, 96, 146,
    218, 312–15
weight loss and, 300–3
blood moles, 130
blouses, 27, 127
body image, 300–315
exercise and, 304–12, 314
posture and, 307, 309–10
weight and, 300–307, 311, 313–14
body temperature, 53, 87, 144
    *see also* fevers
bonding, 199, 203, 208, 211, 237, 247
bottles, bottle feeding, 100, 108
couples and, 271–72
    *see also* formulas, formula feeding
bowel movements, 4, 136, 162–63,
    172–73, 294, 308
childbirth side effects and, 58–61
    *see also* constipation
bras, 21, 26, 127, 170–71, 176, 178–79,
    310
breast-feeding, 6, 21, 26–31, 40, 49–50,
    60, 126–27, 153–93, 299, 301, 310
alternating sides in, 169, 171, 176,
    178, 187
babies feeding enough and, 169, 173
benefits of, 156, 167, 171, 204
breathing and, 50, 165, 170
common myths about, 153–58
c-sections and, 70–71, 76, 164–65
on demand, 163–64
diet and, 135, 137–38, 140–41, 158,
    170, 175, 190–93
emotions and, 153–54, 157–58,
    169–71, 200, 203–5, 212, 218,
    234–35, 240–41, 244, 253, 255
in first week, 161
genital organ care and, 28–31
golden rules of, 161–65

good starts with, 154, 159–84
infections and, 126, 163, 167, 178–79,
    182
latching on and, 165–68, 174, 177
letdown reflex in, 167, 171, 187
lifestyle changes and, 96, 99–100,
    103, 105, 108–9, 111–12
medications and, 70–71, 157, 162,
    176–83, 191
menstrual cycle and, 142–43
positions for, 164–69, 171, 176–77,
    179, 183, 187
postnatal depression and, 231
posture and, 116
problems in, 172–83
reclaiming your body and, 78
routines and, 163, 185–89
sexual intercourse and, 143, 145,
    275–76, 278–79
tips on, 164, 175, 178
work and, 149–50, 158, 185, 188
    *see also* weaning
breast milk, 95, 127, 143–44, 166–67,
    203–4, 212, 240–41
nutritional value of, 157, 163, 166, 190
physical appearance of, 157
production of, 159–61, 172, 180, 187
pumping and storage of, 100, 112,
    143, 149, 158, 169, 171, 174–78,
    183–84, 187–88, 279
treatments and, 14–15, 172, 180
breasts, 20–21, 29, 55, 58, 146
abscesses in, 178–83
acini, 159–60
alveoli, 159–60
areolae, 159, 165, 168, 175–76
body image and, 310–11
before and during breast-feeding, 160
cysts in, 189
engorgement of, 21, 45, 112, 154–55,
    164, 169–70, 173–76, 178–80
physical appearance of, 128, 130, 155
sensitivity of, 161

breasts (*cont'd.*)
　　sizes of, 155, 157, 159, 161, 166, 188, 310
breathing, breathing problems, breathing exercises, 50–51, 111, 119
　　breast-feeding and, 50, 165, 170
　　for childbirth side effects, 53, 57
　　for constipation, 46–47
　　c-sections and, 71–72, 74–76
　　diet and, 138
　　emotions and, 203–4, 227–29, 232
　　genital organ care and, 28–29
　　pelvic floor and, 285, 287–89, 294, 297, 308, 310
　　posture and, 115, 117, 310
　　in reclaiming your body, 81
　　treatments and, 9, 11
　　varicose veins and, 314

calcium, 133
　　breast-feeding and, 190, 192
　　diet and, 135, 137–39
calories, 305
　　breast-feeding and, 190–91, 193
　　diet and, 135, 141
　　weight loss and, 300, 302–3
cardiovascular training, 306–9, 314
carpal tunnel syndrome, 54–55
cars, car seats, 82, 115–16
catheters, 43, 85, 125
　　c-sections and, 69–70, 73
cellulite, 311–12
cervical mucus, 144–45
cervix, 146, 294
　　caring for, 31–32
　　in postpartum complications, 85, 88
　　sexual intercourse and, 274–75, 277, 279
cesarean sections (c-sections), xv, 45, 53–54, 67–77, 82–83, 123–25, 146, 161, 284
　　anesthesia in, 53, 63, 68–71
　　babies born by, 76–77

breast-feeding and, 70–71, 76, 164–65
discomfort after, 70–76
emotions and, 76–77, 201, 207, 212–13
exercises and, 71–72, 74–76, 79, 83, 308
getting out of bed after, 73–74
hygiene and, 74, 121
in postpartum complications, 87, 90
recovery after, 25, 27
scars from, 74, 87, 96, 123–24, 164
sexual intercourse and, 275–77, 279
technique in, 67–69
treatment after, 1, 6, 75
child-bed fever, 85
childbirth, childbirth side effects, 52–66
　　anesthesia and, 53–54, 56–57, 62–66
　　circulatory system and, 53, 57–63
　　common, 52–57
　　emotions in, 206–7
　　pelvic floor and, 287–88, 293
child care, 146, 276
　　couples and, 267, 270–72
　　emotions and, 205–6, 222, 226, 251–56
　　work and, 148–49
childhood, negative aspects of, 248–49
Chinese medicine, xvi, 8–10, 14, 38, 60
chiropractic, 3, 10, 12–13
circulatory problems, 57–58, 90
　　varicose veins, 11, 57, 96, 146, 218, 312–315
classical medications, 1–3, 5–6, 10, 40
coccyx (tailbone), 80, 218
　　childbirth side effects and, 56–57, 64
　　lifestyle changes and, 96
　　pelvic floor and, 285, 289, 299
colostrum, 21, 70, 159–63, 174
combined estrogen/progesterone pills, 144–45
communicating:
　　couples and, 262, 269–71
　　emotions and, 202–5, 210

*Complementary Therapies for Pregnancy and Childbirth* (Tiran and Mack), 6
constipation, 20, 43, 45–49, 59–61, 136, 312
  pelvic floor and, 287–88, 290, 294
  treatment for, 2, 4, 14–15, 46–49, 57, 60–61, 72, 75
contraception, 143–46, 192, 277, 313
cooking:
  diet and, 135, 140
  lifestyle changes and, 101, 103
copper, 24, 131–32, 135, 137
couples, 261–80
  changes in, 261–73
  common stumbling blocks for, 271–72
  emotions and, 209, 262–63, 265–66, 268–69, 277
  father-child relationships and, 268–71
  older, 252
  sexuality and, 263, 267, 274–80
  tips for, 271
  and when men become fathers, 265–68
  and when women become mothers, 262–65
cramps, 111, 113, 122, 232
  diet and, 138
  menstrual cycle and, 142
  treatments for, 54–57, 61
cribs, 106, 109, 114, 223
crying, 143
  breast-feeding and, 154, 163, 171, 173–74
  couples and, 271
  emotions and, 200, 211, 214, 219, 231, 237, 243, 257
  lifestyle changes and, 108
  sexual intercourse and, 276

dairy products, 138–39, 191–92
death, 250–51

depression, 214, 216–25, 234
  breast-feeding and, 157
  causes of, 218–21
  diet and, 136, 138
  exercise and, 120
  fatigue and, 111
  overcoming, 9, 14, 217–25, 230
  symptoms of, 230–32
  work and, 147
  *see also* baby blues; postnatal depression
dermabrasion, 130
diaphragms, 144, 146
diarrhea, 4, 136, 172
diet, diets, xvi, 9, 125–26, 134–41, 155
  basics of, 191–93
  breast-feeding and, 135, 137–38, 140–41, 158, 170, 175, 190–93
  for cellulite, 312
  for childbirth side effects, 60, 62
  for constipation, 46
  couples and, 272
  c-sections and, 71
  digestive system and, 45–46, 136, 139, 141
  emotions and, 217, 219–20, 222–25, 230, 232, 236, 238, 241
  exercise and, 305
  habits and, 139–40
  and how to get what you need, 135–39
  and impact of childbirth, 134–35
  infections and, 125
  lifestyle changes and, 97, 111–12
  physical appearance and, 128
  special needs and, 136–39
  varicose veins and, 314
  for weight loss, 140–41, 158, 272, 300–303, 305, 311
digestive system, 4, 20, 57, 172–73, 211, 295, 302, 308, 312
  breast-feeding and, 156, 163, 167, 173

digestive system (*cont'd.*)
  childbirth side effects and, 53
  c-sections and, 68–72, 75
  diet and, 45–46, 136, 139, 141
  lifestyle changes and, 96
  pelvic floor and, 288
  in postpartum complications, 87
  treatments and, 9, 12–13, 45–49
  *see also* constipation
disappointment, 201, 209
doulas, 103, 189
dream baby, mourning for, 198, 201–2
Dunnewold, Anne, 238

edible oils, 140
elevator exercises, 298
*Emile* (Rousseau), 253
emotional overinvestment, 200
emotions, emotional problems, 146,
    197–258
  bleeding and, 122, 197, 208, 215,
    218–19, 224
  breast-feeding and, 153–54, 157–58,
    169–71, 200, 203–5, 212, 218,
    234–35, 240–41, 244, 253, 255
  in childbirth, 206–7
  child care and, 205–6, 222, 226,
    251–56
  communicating and, 202–5, 210
  couples and, 209, 262–63, 265–66,
    268–69, 277
  c-sections and, 76–77, 201, 207,
    212–13
  exercise and, 78–79, 222, 228, 307–8
  expectations management and, 257–58
  family and, 198, 200–201, 209–10,
    213, 218–19, 227, 233, 235–38,
    244–45, 248–53, 255
  fatigue and, 111, 197–98, 200, 212,
    215, 217–19, 223–24, 226–27, 230,
    232, 234, 236, 238–39, 246–47, 252
  in first days, 197–215
  in first months, 216–32

hormones and, 20–21, 197, 204,
    211–12, 217–19, 226, 235–37, 240,
    244
  and lack of recognition, 255–57
  lifestyle changes and, 96–97, 103–4
  maternal instinct and, 243–44
  mixed, 199–202, 266
  and mother in you, 243–58
  perfectionism and, 220, 244–49, 252,
    255
  posture and, 309
  sexual intercourse and, 232, 246,
    252, 277
  in special cases, 207–11
  in time of change, 197–98
  treatments for, 8–10, 204, 214, 217,
    221, 223–24, 230, 239–42
  weaning and, 189, 240, 251–53
  work and, 148–49, 220–21, 226, 245,
    250, 252–53, 256–57
  in your first encounter with baby,
    199–202
  *see also* baby blues; depression;
    stress; *specific emotions*
epidural catheters, 69
episiotomies, 2, 74, 164
  alternatives to, 34–35
  childbirth side effects and, 58
  emotions and, 211–12
  genital organ care and, 32–41
  hygiene and, 121
  lifestyle changes and, 96
  pain of, 37–41
  pelvic floor and, 286, 289–90, 299
  in postpartum complications, 84, 87
  reclaiming your body and, 79–80
  sexual intercourse and, 275–77,
    279–80, 290
  techniques for, 35
  treatments for, 6, 38–41, 123–24
  urination and, 44
estrogen, 20–21, 44, 59, 90, 111, 131,
    141, 144–45

breast-feeding and, 159–60
emotions and, 211–12, 218, 235
sexual intercourse and, 279
exercise, exercises, xvi, 134, 141
body image and, 304–12, 314
for childbirth side effects, 53–58,
61–62
c-sections and, 71–72, 74–76, 83,
308
digestive system and, 45–49
emotions and, 222, 228, 307–8
for episiotomy pain, 39–41
essential, 119–20
first after childbirth, 49–51
for first six weeks after childbirth,
119–21
how and when to start, 304–5
for pelvic floor, 36, 61, 79–80,
119–21, 285, 288, 293, 295–300,
305, 308
posture and, 120, 307, 309–10
in reclaiming your body, 78–83
varicose veins and, 314
*see also* breathing, breathing
problems, breathing exercises;
relaxation, relaxation exercises
expectations management, 99, 257–58
eyes, 111, 133

family:
breast-feeding and, 154
couples and, 261, 268–70
emotions and, 198, 200–201, 209–10,
213, 218–19, 227, 233, 235–38,
244–45, 248–53, 255
lifestyle changes and, 98, 101–6
work and, 147–48
*see also specific family members*
father, *see couples*
fatigue, 11, 14, 128, 163, 299, 302
breast-feeding and, 158, 179, 186–87
childbirth side effects and, 52–53
couples and, 264–65

diet and, 138, 141
emotions and, 111, 197–98, 200, 212,
215, 217–19, 223–24, 226–27, 230,
232, 234, 236, 238–39, 246–47, 252
genital organ care and, 30
infections and, 125
lifestyle changes and, 95–97, 110–13
recovery process and, 25
sexual intercourse and, 275–76
treatments for, 112–13, 120
fats:
breast-feeding and, 156–58, 167, 191
diet and, 139–41, 303
fears:
couples and, 263–64, 269
sexual intercourse and, 276–77
fertility, fertility treatments, 142–45,
235
fevers, 53, 74
breast-feeding and, 175, 179
infections and, 125
in postpartum complications, 84–87,
89–90
scar healing and, 123
fiber, 139
Fitzgerald, William, 14
Fletcher, Gillian, 98–99
fluid intake, 45–46
breast-feeding and, 170, 187, 191
childbirth side effects and, 53–54
for constipation, 46, 48
infections and, 125
fluid retention, 26, 44–45, 141, 156,
311–12
breast-feeding and, 163
childbirth side effects and, 54–55
c-sections and, 69
exercises and, 49
forceps deliveries, 63, 201, 275
emotions and, 207, 213
formulas, formula feeding, 185
comparisons between breast-feeding
and, 156, 173

formulas, formula feeding (*cont'd.*)
  cow's milk, 153, 156
  supplementing breast-feeding with,
    172–75, 187
Freud, Sigmund, 254, 263
friends:
  breast-feeding and, 154, 161
  couples and, 265, 267–68
  emotions and, 198, 200, 209–10,
    213, 218–19, 223–24, 227, 233, 252,
    257
  lifestyle changes and, 101, 103–6,
    109
fruits, 137–40, 192, 302

garlic, 175
gas, gas pain, 45, 79, 120, 136, 192
  c-sections and, 71–72, 76
  pelvic floor and, 288, 290, 293–94
  treatments for, 47–48, 72, 76
Gattefosse, Rene Maurice, 7
genetics:
  emotions and, 235, 243
  varicose veins and, 313–14
genital organs, genital organ care,
    22–23, 28–41, 45, 120–21, 128
  birth canal and, 31–33
  childbirth side effects and, 57
  episiotomies and, 32–41
  hygiene and, 43, 121
  infections of, 32, 36–38, 84–85, 87
  lifestyle changes and, 96
  menstrual cycle and, 142–45
  pelvic floor and, 284–85, 288–89, 2
    94
  sexual intercourse and, 274–75
  uterus and, 28–31
good-enough mothers, 246–47
grains, 137–39, 224–25
grandmothers:
  emotions and, 205, 220, 237, 245,
    248–51, 257
  help from, 102, 104, 112

growth spurts, 186, 211
  lifestyle changes and, 99–100
gums, 132–33

Hahnemann, Samuel, 4
hair:
  appearance of, 127–28, 131–32
  loss of, 219, 232
Hamilton, James, 198
headaches, xiv, 53–54, 64, 90, 219, 225,
    232
heartburn, 11, 45, 111
help:
  emotions and, 205, 217, 222–23, 230
  fatigue and, 112
  right kind of, 101–4
hematomas, 32, 79
hemorrhages, 88–89
hemorrhoids, xiii, 46, 58–62, 70, 111,
    138, 212, 218, 294
  causes of, 59
  lifestyle changes and, 96
  treatment of, 11, 15, 60–62
herbal remedies, 2–3, 6–8, 10
  for after-pains, 30
  for baby blues, 215
  for body toning, 311
  for breast milk production, 172
  for chapped nipples, 182
  for childbirth side effects, 59–61
  for constipation, 48
  for c-sections, 75
  for depression, 225
  for engorgement, 180
  for episiotomy pain, 40
  for fatigue, 113
  for hair, 131
  for infections, 127
  for mastitis, 179
  for menstrual cycle, 143
  for organ prolapses, 295
  for postpartum complications, 86, 90
  in recovery process, 24, 27

for vaginal area, 36
for weight loss, 302
Hill, Christine, 98, 100
homeopathy, xvi, 2–6, 8, 239, 241
   for after-pains, 30
   for baby blues, 215
   for bleeding, 122
   for breast abscesses, 182
   for breast milk production, 172, 180
   for childbirth side effects, 54, 56, 59,
      61, 64
   for constipation, 48
   for c-sections, 75
   for depression, 225
   for engorgement, 180
   for episiotomy pain, 40
   for fatigue, 113
   for mastitis, 182
   for menstrual cycle, 143
   for organ prolapses, 295
   for pain during breast-feeding, 181
   for postpartum complications, 86–87
   in recovery process, 24, 27
   for scar healing, 124
   for vaginal area, 36
   for weight loss, 302
hormones, 19–21, 89, 310–13
   body toning and, 310–12
   breast-feeding and, 154–55, 159–62,
      169–71, 175
   childbirth side effects and, 52, 59
   after delivery, 21
   diet and, 138–39, 141
   emotions and, 20–21, 197, 204,
      211–12, 217–19, 226, 235–37, 240,
      244
   lifestyle changes and, 96
   menstrual cycle and, 143
   pelvic floor and, 284, 288, 294, 296,
      299
   physical appearance and, 128–29,
      131–32
   during pregnancy, 20

reclaiming your body and, 79–80
   sexual intercourse and, 275, 279
   varicose veins and, 313
hospitals, 107
   environment of, 214
   hygiene in, 43
   tips for calm departure from, 82–83
   what to bring to, 26–27
housekeeping:
   couples and, 265, 272
   emotions and, 202
   lifestyle changes and, 100–103
   posture and, 118
husbands, xv–xvi, 69, 146
   breast-feeding and, 161–62
   emotions and, 198–203, 205, 210–11,
      213, 219, 221–24, 227, 232–33,
      236–37, 246–47, 249–50, 252, 254,
      256
   exercise and, 304
   lifestyle changes and, 98–99, 101–2,
      107, 109
   see also couples
hygiene:
   breast-feeding and, 171, 174, 176–77
   c-sections and, 74, 121
   infections and, 43, 121, 126
   lifestyle changes and, 109
   in postpartum complications, 84–85,
      87
   scar healing and, 123
   for teeth, 133

immune system, 10, 140, 156
   diet and, 136
   emotions and, 227
   in postpartum complications, 86
indifference, 200
infections, 1, 53, 121–27, 292, 298
   bleeding and, 122
   breast-feeding and, 126, 163, 167,
      178–79, 182
   c-sections and, 69–70, 74

infections (*cont'd.*)
emotions and, 204, 227
genital organ care and, 32, 36–38,
84–85, 87
hygiene and, 43, 121, 126
as postpartum complications, 84–89
scar healing and, 123
sexual intercourse and, 126, 277, 280
Ingham, Eunice, 14
insomnia, 113, 295
coping with, 222–23
emotions and, 230, 239
intrauterine devices (IUDs), 144
intravenous (IV) tubes, xv
c-sections and, 69–70, 73–74
for postpartum complications, 87, 89
iron, 53, 58, 135–37, 219

Kegel exercises, 80, 296
kidneys, 9, 124–25, 156, 211, 291
infections of, 86–87
Kitzinger, Sheila, 237

lactation consultants, 103, 153, 161, 172
laxatives, 2, 49, 60–61, 139, 162
Leboyer, Frédéric, 204, 208
lecithin, 224
legs, 54, 310–11, 315
letdown reflex, 167, 171, 187
lifestyle, lifestyle changes, 95–113, 312,
314
childbirth side effects, 61–62
fatigue and, 95–97, 110–13
fragile body and, 95–97
organizing your return home and,
100–104
relationship changes and, 104–9
routines for, 97–100, 106, 108,
110–11, 113
liposuction, 131, 312
lochia, 23, 121–22, 136
lifestyle changes and, 96, 102
in postpartum complications, 85, 89

loneliness, 186, 198, 221, 236, 265
lying down:
breast-feeding and, 164, 166
childbirth side effects and, 56
c-sections and, 71–73, 76
emotions and, 229
exercises and, 49–51, 57, 62, 297,
308–9
in genital organ care, 29
lifestyle changes and, 97, 112
posture in, 117
reclaiming your body and, 79–83

Mack, Sue, 6
magnesium, 135, 137–39
manual therapies, xvi, 10–15
Marcé, L. V., 216
massages, 3, 7, 10, 14, 117, 184, 311
breast-feeding and, 170, 177
for chapped nipples, 181
for childbirth side effects, 53–57
for constipation, 47–49
emotions and, 204, 224
pelvic floor and, 288, 296
for scar healing, 124
sexual intercourse and, 278
for skin, 129, 131
for uterus, 29–31
mastitis, 178–79, 182
maternity clothes, 82, 127
Maury, Marguerite, 7
meats, 192, 224, 302, 312
diet and, 136–37, 139
meconium, 162–63
medical teams, reactions toward, 210
medications, 31, 82
bleeding and, 122–23
breast-feeding and, 70–71, 157, 162,
176–83, 191
childbirth side effects and, 53–54,
56–58, 60–66
classical, 1–3, 5–6, 10, 40
in c-sections, 68–71, 74

digestive system and, 46, 49
emotions and, 217, 230, 239–42
infections and, 125–26
menstrual cycle and, 142
for postpartum complications, 85–87,
    89–90
scar healing and, 123
side effects of, 1–2, 68–69, 71,
    240–41
for skin outbreaks, 130
for urinary incontinence, 292
*see also* anesthesia
menopause, 253, 284, 292, 294, 313
menstrual cycle, 23, 122, 128, 141–46,
    219, 279, 299, 310
diet and, 136
fertility and, 142–45
and first period after childbirth,
    142–43
resumption of, 142–45
teeth and, 133
minerals:
breast-feeding and, 163, 166
diet and, 134–39
in recovery process, 24
mineral water, 27, 39, 138–39
mini-pills, 144–45
monoamine oxidase (MAO), 212
mood swings, 211, 268
morphine, 6, 53, 68–71
mothers:
physical appearance of, 126–33
self-perceptions of, 257
mothers-in-law, 276
emotions and, 227, 248–51
help from, 102, 104
multiple pregnancies, 207–8
musculoskeletal system, 20, 113, 127
breast-feeding and, 164
childbirth side effects and, 54–57, 63,
    66
contraception and, 144
in c-sections, 68, 71–72, 74–76

diet and, 138–39, 303
digestive system and, 45, 47
emotions and, 227–28
exercise and, 79–83, 304, 306–10, 312
genital organ care and, 30, 32–33, 35
lifestyle changes and, 96
posture and, 115–17, 309
recovery process and, 25
sexual intercourse and, 275, 280
treatments and, 9, 11, 13, 79–83
*see also specific muscles and bones*

nails, 128, 132
naps, 223, 227–28, 230
*see also* sleep
narcotic analgesics, 1–2, 6, 46, 53, 68–71
natural contraceptive methods, 144
nausea and vomiting, 11, 53, 69–70,
    136, 172, 252
nerves, nervous system, 141
breast-feeding and, 191–92
emotions and, 203–4
genital organ care and, 35
treatments and, 9, 11, 13–14
*New Mother's Body Book* (Shannon), 257
nightgowns, 26, 44
nightmares, 111, 230, 267
nipples, 159–60, 162, 176–79, 183–84,
    199
artificial, 172
injuries to, 164, 167–69, 176–79,
    181–82
in latching on, 165–68, 174, 177
nonsteroidal anti-inflammatory drugs
    (NSAIDs), 1, 31, 40
numbness, 200, 234
nuts, 137–39, 192, 224–25

obstetricians, 3, 103, 146, 289
childbirth side effects and, 63
in c-sections, 68
episiotomies and, 33–35, 38
overemphasizing role of, 264

older mothers, 252–53

organ prolapses:
  causes of, 293–94
  genital organ care and, 33–34
  pelvic floor and, 284, 293–95, 298, 308
  treatment for, 294–95
  warning signs of, 294

osteopathy, 3, 10–13, 239, 241

oxytocin, 1–2, 21, 25, 29, 68, 89, 122, 279, 289
  breast-feeding and, 160, 162, 170–71


pain:
  abdominal, 85, 125
  after a cesarean, 70–71
  emotions and, 218–19
  of episiotomies, 37–41
  pelvic floor and, 289–90, 294–95
  sexual intercourse and, 276, 279–80, 290, 294–95
  treatments for, 54–57, 61, 181
  see also gas, gas pain

Palmer, Daniel, 13

pantothenic acid (vitamin B₅), 224

Pap smears, 146

partner, see couples

pediatricians, 82
  emotions and, 239, 246–47, 254, 256
  posture and, 116
  selection of, 103–4

pelvic balance:
  exercises for, 119–20
  recovery of, 80–83

pelvic floor, pelvic floor muscles, 29, 32, 283–300
  anus and, 284–86, 293, 297–98
  exercises for, 36, 61, 79–80, 119–21, 285, 288, 293, 295–300, 305, 308
  factors impacting on, 287–90
  importance of, 283–85
  lifestyle changes and, 96
  myths about, 284

organ prolapses and, 284, 293–95, 298, 308

posture and, 115–16, 284, 287, 296, 310

during pregnancy, 287–88, 296

urinary incontinence and, 283–84, 287–88, 290–99

urogenital problems and, 290–91, 295

pelvis, 56, 64
  anatomy of, 285–86

perfectionism:
  couples and, 270, 272
  emotions and, 220, 244–49, 252, 255

perineal massage, 288, 296

perineum, 15, 47, 120, 146
  childbirth side effects and, 58, 61
  contraception and, 144
  genital organ care and, 32–39
  in postpartum complications, 84, 86–87
  urination and, 43

perioral dermatitis, 130

pets, 109

phlebitis, 58, 90

phlegm, 71–72

physical therapy, 298–99

placenta, 20–23, 53, 58, 160, 244
  bleeding and, 122–23
  c-sections and, 68
  emotions and, 211–12
  hormones and, 20–21
  in postpartum complications, 88–90
  recovery process and, 23, 25
  reproductive system and, 22

postnatal depression, 97, 145, 198, 210, 216–17, 221, 230–42, 252, 275
  causes of, 235–38
  consequences of, 237–38
  diagnosis of, 238–39
  hormones and, 21
  predisposition to, 234–35
  symptoms of, 217, 230–32, 233–35, 238–40
  treatments for, 217, 230, 237–42

postnatal visits, 145–46
postpartum complications, 84–91
　blood and bleeding as, 84–85, 87–90
　infections as, 84–89
posture, xvi, 114–18
　in bed, 117
　body image and, 307, 309–10
　childbirth side effects and, 56
　exercise and, 120, 307, 309–10
　at home, 116–18
　lifestyle changes and, 96–97
　pelvic floor and, 115–16, 284, 287,
　　296, 310
　when caring for babies, 114–16
potassium, deficiency in, 219
pregnancy masks, 128
pregnancy tumor, 132
premature babies:
　breast-feeding of, 174, 183–84
　emotions and, 207–8, 211
privacy, 278
progesterone, 20, 45, 132, 141
　breast-feeding and, 159–60
　emotions and, 212, 218, 235–36
progesterone mini-pills, 144–45
prolactin, 21, 141, 159–61, 169, 175,
　204, 212, 275
　emotions and, 235, 244
proteins:
　breast-feeding and, 156, 163, 166,
　　191
　diet and, 135, 137, 139, 303, 312
psychotherapy, 239, 241–42
puerperal psychosis, 217
　symptoms of, 234, 242
　treatment of, 230, 242

recovery process, 23–27
recreation, 221, 223
rectum, see anus
reflexology, 3, 14–15
regrets, 212–13
relationship changes, 104–9

relaxation, relaxation exercises, 15, 256
　for childbirth side effects, 53–54
　couples and, 267
　c-sections and, 74
　emotions and, 221, 227–30, 239–41,
　　253
　in genital organ care, 29
　pelvic floor and, 296–97
　positions for, 229
　posture and, 309
resentment, 209
rest, 134
　breast-feeding and, 176, 178
　emotions and, 214, 221, 223, 230
　lifestyle changes and, 97, 100
Rousseau, Jean-Jacques, 253
routines:
　breast-feeding and, 163, 185–89
　couples and, 269
　emotions and, 198, 238
　for lifestyle changes, 97–100, 106,
　　108, 110–11, 113
　running, 305

salad dressings, 140
salts, 134, 140, 311–12
　breast-feeding and, 163, 166
Sanford, Diane, 238
sanitary napkins, 82–83
sclerotherapy, 315
seafood, 137–39, 192, 224, 302, 312
selective serotonin reuptake inhibitors
　(SSRIs), 240
self, fear of losing, 200, 221
sexuality, sexual intercourse, 70
　contraception and, 143–46, 192, 277,
　　313
　couples and, 263, 267, 274–80
　emotions and, 232, 246, 252, 277
　episiotomies and, 38, 275–77,
　　279–80, 290
　infections and, 126, 277, 280
　pelvic floor and, 285, 288–90, 294–95

sexuality, sexual intercourse (*cont'd.*)
  physical impediments to, 274–75
  psychological impediments to,
    275–76
  reclaiming intimacy and, 277–80
  transitional, 277–78
shame, 209
Shannon, Jacqueline, 257
shiatsu/acupressure, 3, 9–10, 13–14
shivers and trembling, 53
shopping, 100–101, 103–4, 223
shoulders, 288
  breast-feeding and, 170
  c-sections and, 70
  emotions and, 228–29
  posture and, 116–17, 309
siblings, 187, 256, 278
  before delivery, 106–7
  emotions and, 238
  lifestyle changes and, 98, 101, 103,
    106–9, 111–12
  when you come home, 107–9
  while you are in hospital, 107
sick babies:
  breast-feeding for, 183–84
  emotions and, 208–10
single mothers, 203
sitting:
  breast-feeding and, 164–66
  c-sections and, 73, 76
  emotions and, 228–29
  posture in, 116–17
sitz baths, 60
skin, 70–71, 140
  acne and, 70, 128, 130
  appearance of, 127–31
  breast-feeding and, 155, 171, 178
  c-sections and, 68, 71, 74
  emotions and, 203–4, 208
  infections and, 125–26
  itching and, 71, 74, 111, 125–26, 138
  pigmentation and, 96
  stretch marks on, 130–31, 155

skin tabs, 130
sleep, 11, 19, 52, 239, 295, 301
  breast-feeding and, 154, 162–64,
    169–70, 173–75, 183, 186–87
  couples and, 271
  diet and, 138
  emotions and, 198, 211–13, 218, 220,
    222–23, 226–28, 230, 234, 237, 242
  exercise and, 120
  in genital organ care, 29
  lack of, 110–11, 141, 218, 223
  lifestyle changes and, 99–100, 107–8,
    110–13
slippers, 26
smoking, 116, 191
Snuglis®, 115
specialists, 238–39
spermicides, 144–45
spine, 285
  childbirth side effects and, 54, 64
  c-sections and, 69
  manual therapies and, 10–13
  *see also* back, back pain
standing, 71, 73–74
star angiomas, 130
status, loss of, 200, 213–14
Still, Andrew Taylor, 11
stress, 15, 197, 202–3, 214, 224–29, 256
  breast-feeding and, 157
  diet and, 138
  fatigue and, 111–12
  lifestyle changes and, 98–99
  management of, 226–29
  physical signs of, 227
  postnatal depression and, 236–37
  in response to situations, 227
  symptoms of, 246
stress incontinence, 96, 292
stretch marks, 130–31, 155
suffocation, feeling of, 263
sugar, sugars, 312
  breast-feeding and, 157–58, 163, 193
  diet and, 140–41

infections and, 125
superwomen, 98–100
support networks, 103–4
surgery, 81, 86, 183, 293–95
  for childbirth side effects, 62
  for organ prolapses, 294–95
  for urinary incontinence, 293
  for varicose veins, 315
  *see also specific procedures*
Sutherland, William Garner, 11
swimming, 305–7

tears, 32–33
teeth, 132–33, 138
tennis, 305
tension, tensions, 209–10, 227–29, 245–49
  couples and, 263, 270
  depression and, 225
  family and, 248–49
  perfectionism and, 245–46
  postnatal depression and, 236
  stress and, 228–29
thighs, toning of, 311
Thomas, Patricia, 3–4
Thoracic Outlet Syndrome, 55
thrombosis, 58, 90
thrush, 127
thyroid malfunction, 219
Tiran, Denise, 6
toys, 107–8, 245, 254
trace elements, 134, 136–37
tranquilizers, 240

uncertainty, 212–13
urethra, 34, 64, 124–25
  c-sections and, 69–70
  pelvic floor and, 284–86, 289, 291
  urination and, 42
urinary incontinence, xiv, 92, 218, 252, 280
  genital organ care and, 33–34
  pelvic floor and, 283–84, 287–88, 290–99

treatment for, 292–93
urinary tract infections (cystitis), 85–87, 124–25
  c-sections and, 69–70
  treatments for, 1, 12, 86–87
urine, urination, 42–45, 146, 294
  breast-feeding and, 173
  childbirth side effects and, 64
  c-sections and, 70
  genital organ care and, 37
  induction of, 43–44
  reclaiming your body and, 83
  stopping in midstream, 79, 120, 297–98
  weight loss and, 301
urogenital system, urogenital problems, 20, 290–91, 295
  *see also* genital organs, genital organ care
uterine atony, 88
uterus, 19–25, 45, 55, 144–46, 162, 204
  bleeding and, 88–89, 122–23
  breast-feeding and, 170
  caring for, 28–31
  childbirth side effects and, 57–59
  contraception and, 144–45
  coping with after-pains of, 28–31
  in c-sections, 68, 70–71, 74
  exercise and, 309
  hormones and, 20–21
  infections of, 85, 88
  pelvic floor and, 286–89, 294, 296
  reclaiming your body and, 80
  recovery process and, 23–25
  sexual intercourse and, 275, 277
  treatments and, 1–2, 6, 11, 15, 29–31
  in urination, 42
  varicose veins and, 313

vagina, 70, 80, 120, 313–14
  caring for, 31–33, 35–36
  contraception and, 144
  discharges from, 84, 89, 125–26

vagina (*cont'd.*)
  infections of, 84–85, 124–26
  pelvic floor and, 284–86, 289–90,
    294, 297–99
  sexual intercourse and, 275–76,
    278–80, 289–90
varicose veins, 11, 57, 96, 146, 218,
    312–15
vegetables, 135–39, 192–93, 224–25,
    302
visitors, 170, 214
  lifestyle changes and, 105–6, 109
vitamins, 134–40
  A, 61, 130, 171, 192
  B, 131–32, 135–38, 192, 224, 275,
    302, 314
  C, 135, 137, 179
  D, 61, 138
  E, 61, 171, 225, 302
  emotions and, 224–25, 239
vulva, 280, 286, 294, 298
  childbirth side effects and, 57
  genital organ care and, 32–33, 36

walking, 49–50, 228, 305–7, 314
  for childbirth side effects, 58
  c-sections and, 69, 73–74, 82
  one hour each day, 120
  posture and, 116, 309
water, 27, 39, 138–39, 167
  *see also* fluid intake; fluid retention
weaning, 131–32, 188–89, 310
  emotions and, 189, 240, 251–53
  of siblings, 107

weight, 113, 134, 252, 275
  body image and, 300–307, 311,
    313–14
  breast-feeding and, 156, 158, 163,
    187, 190–91
  childbirth side effects and, 53, 55, 57
  couples and, 272
  exercise and, 304–7
  goals for, 301–3
  lifestyle changes and, 96
  loss of, 140–41, 158, 272, 300–307, 311
  manual therapies and, 10–11
  postnatal visits and, 146
  posture and, 115–16
  varicose veins and, 313–14
Winnicott, Donald, 199, 247
witch hazel, 36–37, 40, 60–61, 71
work:
  breast-feeding and, 149–50, 158, 185,
    188
  couples and, 263, 266–68
  emotions and, 148–49, 220–21, 226,
    245, 250, 252–53, 256–57
  lifestyle changes and, 104
  pelvic floor and, 298
  returning to, 147–50, 188
  sexual intercourse and, 276

yeast infections, 125–27

zinc, 192, 225, 302
  diet and, 135, 137
  for hair, 128, 131–32